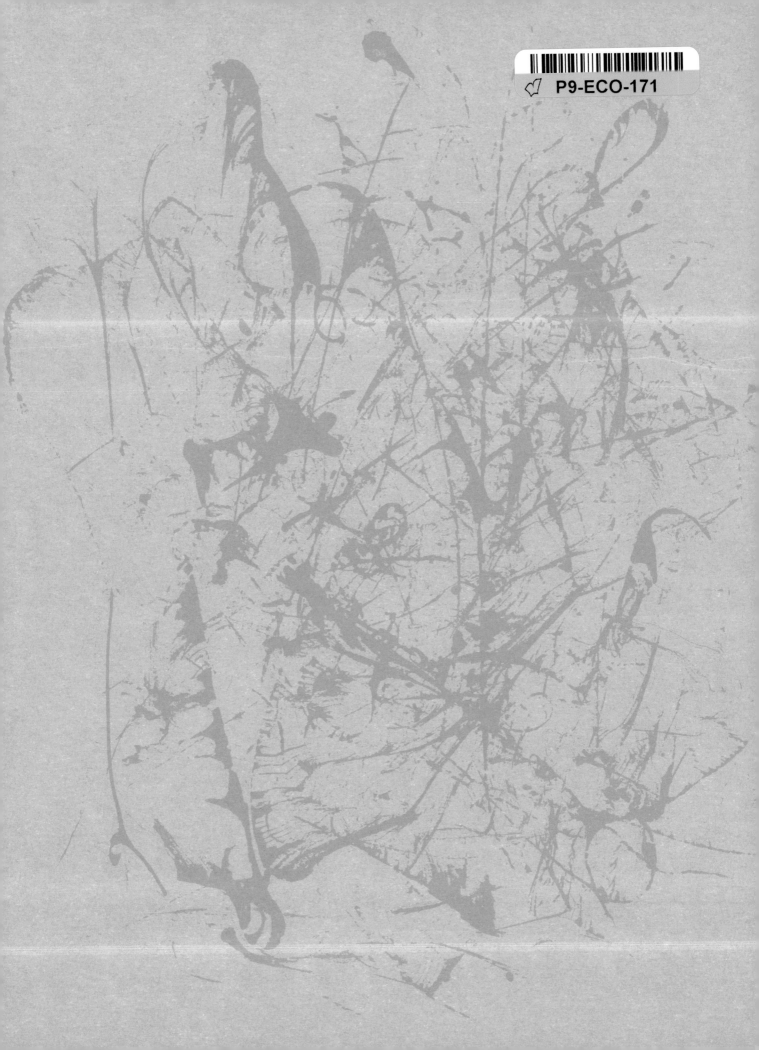

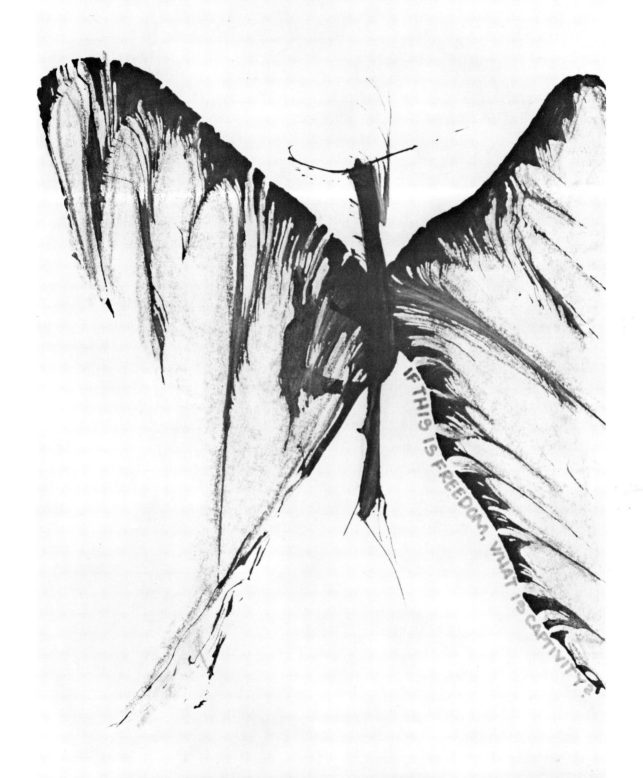

IF THIS IS FREEDOM, WHAT IS CAPTIVITY?

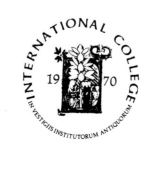

The Guild of Tutors Press

1019 Gayley Avenue   Los Angeles, California 90024

(213) 477-6761

a
compilation
of
feelings
by

RIGHT BRAIN PEOPLE IN A LEFT BRAIN WORLD

as expressed to **EVELYN VIRSHUP**
m.a., a.t.r.

through art as therapy

An ART THERAPY WEST Book

Chapters of this book have been adapted from a series of
articles which appeared in ARTS AND ACTIVITIES, 1978.

RIGHT-LEFT BRAIN artwork appeared originally in
IN TOUCH THROUGH ART, by Eslinger, Virshup,
and Arrington, 1976

National Gallery of Art has granted permission to reproduce
the artwork by M. C. Escher and E. Munch.

**GRAPHIC DESIGN BY
BERNARD CLENDENIN AND EVELYN VIRSHUP**

Library of Congress Catalog Card Number 78-69852

Virshup, Evelyn
RIGHT BRAIN PEOPLE IN A LEFT BRAIN WORLD

Includes bibliography and index
Contents:
1. Drug Addicts' and alcoholics' drawings.
2. Art therapy concepts and exercises.

(Hardcover) ISBN 89615-042-9

(Paperback) ISBN 89615-043-7

DEDICATION

To the RIGHT BRAIN people of our world

who were told at an early age that

they had no "artistic talent" . . . . .

they shouldn't waste their time

daydreaming and fantasizing . . . . .

they shouldn't trust their intuition . . . . .

they should be rational and logical

at all times . . . . .

to those people, who undervalue their

imagery, I dedicate this book.

"I cannot forbear to mention. . . a new device for study which, although it may seem trivial and almost ludicrous, is nevertheless extremely useful in arousing the mind to various inventions. And this is, when you look at a wall spotted with stains. . . you may discover a resemblance to various landscapes, beautified with mountains, rivers, rocks, trees. . . or again you may see battles and figures in action, or strange faces and costumes and an endless variety of objects which you could reduce to complete and well-drawn forms. And these appear on such walls confusedly, like the sound of bells in whose jangle you may find any name or word you choose to imagine.

"

Leonardo da Vinci

ACHNOWLEDGEMENTS

I give thanks to the people who helped me begin to understand the language of art: Marvin Harden, who made me stay with my drawings until they were a part of me; Virginia Rothman, who helped me forget the product for the process; Dorothy Royer and Toby Reisel, who encouraged me to organize and articulate my many simultaneous and diffusely focused thoughts on art therapy; Sue Anne Eslinger, whose energy and enthusiasm for putting it all together in book form, mobilized me; and especially to my clients (whose book this is).

I give many thanks to Bernie Clendenin, whose graphic vision and patience brought into reality the vision in my mind's eye, and Lynda Marin, who labored over my manuscript helping to make it orderly, sequential and rational. Al Muscatel and his staff gave of their time and support for the art therapy program at Tarzana Psychiatric Hospital. Lynn Martin Chusid, generously allowed me to reproduce some of her beautiful collection of graphics and sculpture.

And finally, my thanks to my mother, Estelle Weinstock, my sons, David, Gary and Steven, and my husband and best friend, Bernie, who all supported me emotionally as I struggled to learn about myself through the language of art.

8

contents

FOREWORD

The age of reason was ushered in with the statement, "I think, therefore I am." Logic and science with precision and direction cleared the air of the miasma of superstition and unfounded beliefs which had shackled man's progress to the pronouncements of oracles and priests of centuries before. Mathematics, physics and chemistry explored the molecule, energy and the universe; medicine and psychology developed a rational basis. The benefits were enormous in the power and scope of mankind's achievements.

And yet, was there something which was lost? Or at least ignored, passed over? Something vague, insubstantial, not clearly understood, and yet pervasively referred to by artists, poets, musicians and mystics?

In the last few years, a new story has been developing with implications that touch the lives of every one of us.

After the first world war, there were some amusing clinical anecdotes of people with selective left cerebral hemisphere injuries who were aphasic, and couldn't think straight, but who nevertheless functioned, in an inadequate sort of way, with feelings and concepts that they couldn't quite express.

And we have all known people with left-sided cerebral strokes whose eyes followed us, with speechless frustration, at not being able to express something.

But then, in 1964, Bogen and Sperry and their associates began to investigate this phenomenon in patients whose corpus callosum, the connection between the left and right hemisphere, was surgically cut to help control their epilepsy. Their findings of really significant differences in the two hemispheres opened the way for a new understanding of these neglected and abused functions.

One clear fact evolved; the right brain, with all its valuable attributes, is just not very verbal, and in ease of communication and expression, it loses hands down to its verbal, logical, sequential mate.

But what has also evolved, is that the right brain is visual and can easily conceptualize and communicate with images. Of course, artists have been doing this for aeons. But somehow, it seems as though the right brain has been talking only to the right brain, and there has been something missing, a gap.

And now, in what I can only describe as a breakthrough, Evelyn describes a means of integrating the two sides of the brain, in a manner so simple, yet so elegant, that leads one to say, "Of course! Why didn't anyone do it this way before?"

In this book she describes and graphically illustrates the process of projecting an image, and then "gestalting" the result. That is, she describes the process by which people can draw their mental images onto paper (and in the text she describes many different ways of accomplishing this), and then, as the object they have drawn, they describe themselves in words.

She describes this process in words which are useful to art therapists, students, teachers, those dealing with drug addicts, or any other addiction, and in fact to anyone in the helping professions. But even of more importance, she is careful to describe the process in words which make it useful for any individual, for anyone interested in self-awareness and growth.

But the major part of the book, the drawings and words created by her drug addict clients, speak for themselves in a new language, with poignancy and clarity. The demonstration of the ease with which these inarticulate people could communicate their feelings of frustration, inadequacy and pain, when given the proper tools, must stand as a milestone in man's understanding of himself.

No longer need the depth and richness of the right brain's contribution to life be ignored or deprecated because of the left brain's ease of expression through language; it must step forward to take its proper, long denied place as an equal partner in man's progress toward — where? Its future seems as rich and varied, in relief of pain and addiction, in holistic healing, in self awareness and growth, as imagination itself.

So never think for one moment that this book is only about drug addicts. It is about, and for, YOU.

Bernard B. Virshup, M.D.

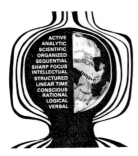

Active
Analytic
Scientific
Organized
Sequential
Sharp Focus
Intellectual
Structured
Linear Time
Conscious
Rational
Logical
Verbal

INTRODUCTION

For a year, I worked as an art therapist at a residential rehabilitation center for drug abusers. The artwork following was done by the young men and women hospitalized there. None of them had any formal art training.

METHOD

At each session, I provided kite string which the patients soaked in ink and dragged across the paper, making abstract designs. Then they turned the paper around sideways and upside down until they found some image they could develop with pastels and felt-tipped pens, bringing their images more into focus. When they had done this, I would ask them to write stories or poems about their drawings, and then read them to the group, if they wished.

PROCESS AND PERCEPTION

I believe that all the marks we make on paper, all the colors and gestures we choose to use, are extensions of thoughts and feelings going on inside of ourselves. Therefore, our drawings and what we write about them are, in a very real sense, a description of how we perceive ourselves on an unconscious level. By drawing this way, we are able to make our unconscious more conscious. As Freud described dreaming, drawing is another "royal road to the unconscious."

BRAIN INTEGRATION

Another concept of the art therapy process is that it integrates the functions of the right and left hemisphere of the brain. Art is visual, imaginative and intuitive thinking; these are right brain functions. The ability to create a logical, orderly, sequential narrative about the art process is a left brain function. I consider it important that people whose dominant mode of function is either right or left, learn to integrate the functions of the opposite side.

RISKS

Because the drawing was spontaneous and not product-oriented, the patients' anxieties about showing their "lack of talent" was lessened, and they were more comfortable with sharing their work. In this atmosphere, they were willing to take more risks, and be more expressive.

MASKS AND MANNERISMS

Drug addicts, even as you and I, have many thoughts and feelings they have not been able to tell anyone. They have developed masks and mannerisms covering up their feelings of inadequacy, shame and isolation. Through their artwork in the group, they found themselves drawing and saying things they had never admitted to anyone before. As they drew more pictures in which they saw themselves and their feelings, these untutored artists were able to gradually and graphically express their long pent-up anguish, confusion, rage and frustration.

FEELINGS

The other members of the groups were very accepting of these powerful feelings because they felt the same way. Feelings of closeness and trust, and the ability to be more open and accepting of themselves and others developed as they shared their humiliations and anger in our art therapy sessions.

The feelings their artwork has shown are universal.

This commonality bonds us together in the human condition.

13

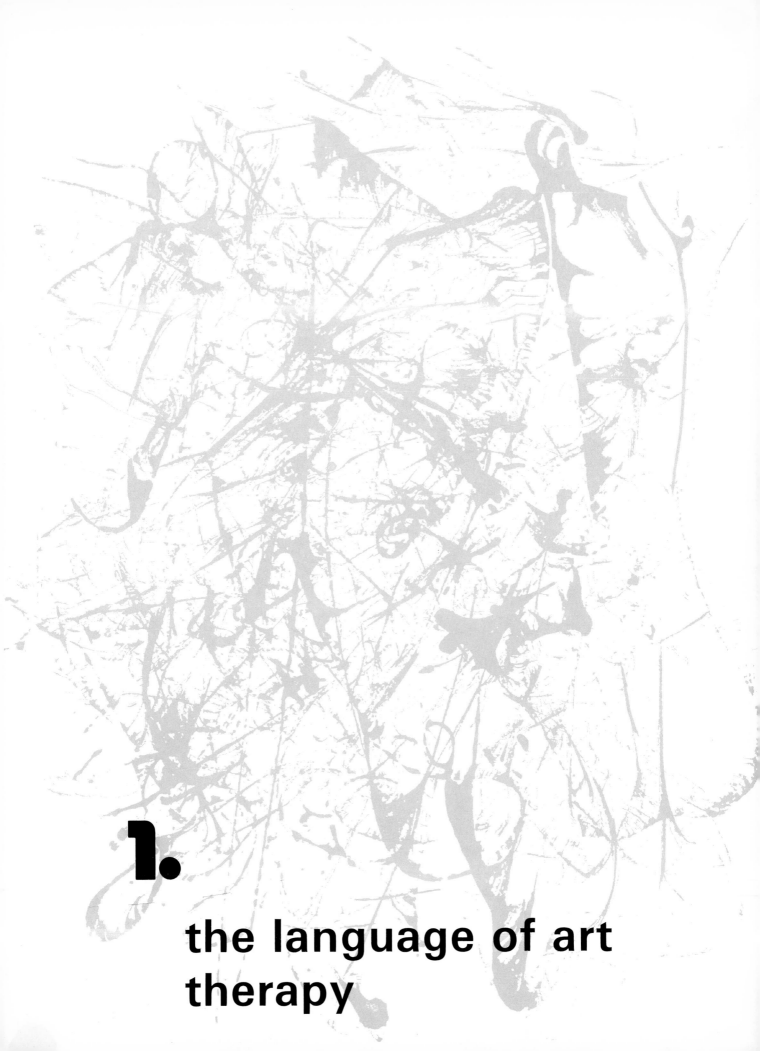

1.

the language of art therapy

"This is a man
hiding behind a mask,
who doesn't know how to
show his real face."

The clown's mask not
only hides the man's
identity, but shows
that he does not take
himself seriously, or
think that he is worthwhile.

16

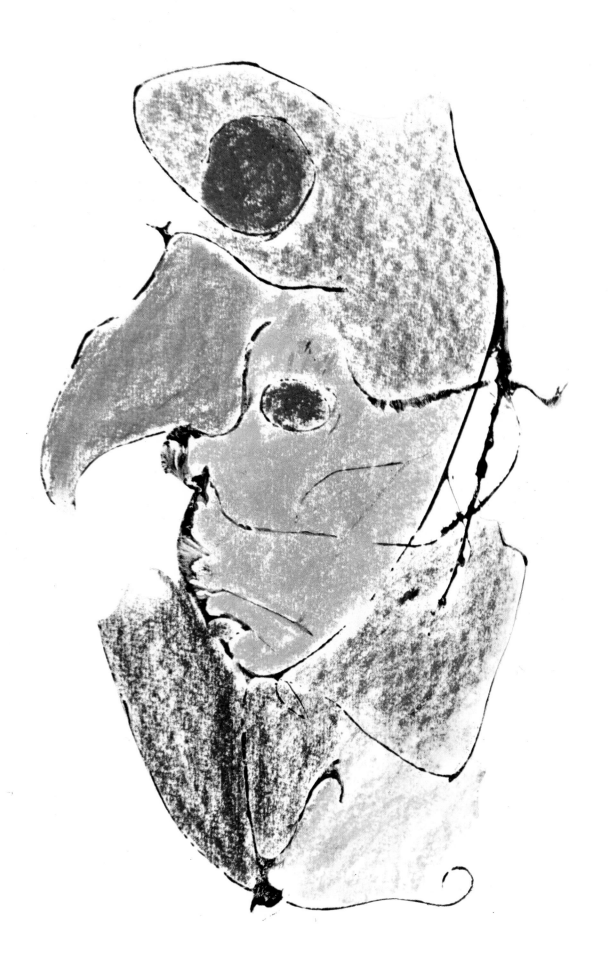

17

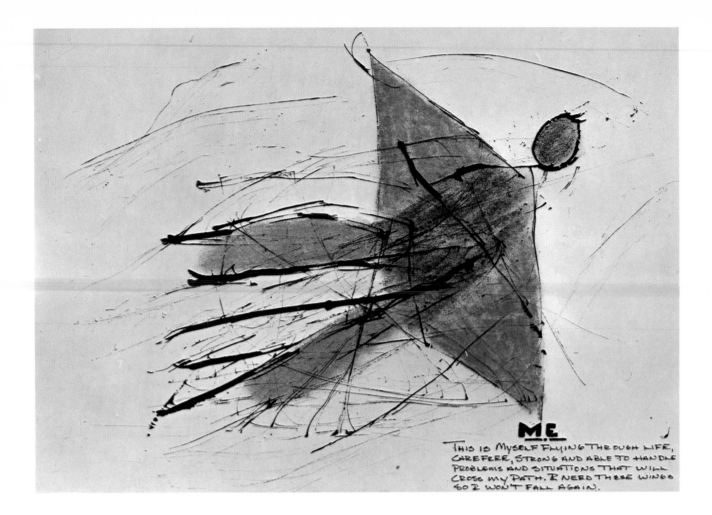

This is Myself flying through life, carefree, strong and able to handle problems and situations that will cross my path. I need these wings so I won't fall again.

TED, a self-described con-man and former musician started using drugs at age 14 to belong to a gang. He gave up his music, and began dealing instead.

His statement, Me, conflicts with his drawing. His "carefree and strong" self has no eyes or ears to recognize his problems, his lack of hands and feet prevented him from resolving them, and his colorful wings help him avoid them.

Art therapy, using art as another language, is a way of allowing people to understand themselves, their conflicts, and their relationships, through drawing, sculpting, and painting.

The process has been clarified by recent "split-brain" research which has clearly shown that the ability to create a logical, orderly narrative can be differentiated from the imaginative, holistic intuitive functions that are primary in art and fantasy.

Although split-brain research has anatomically localized these functions into each hemisphere, it has been accurately pointed out that the unsplit brain normally integrates these functions so that each half deals with both, more or less simultaneously. Indeed, an important function of art therapy is to improve just this type of integrated communication.

Carl Jung wrote about this concept many years ago, before localization was known, in his discussion of psychological types. He described four modes of looking at the world; thinking, feeling, sensation and intuition. The thinking mode was logical and ordered (cogito, ergo sum). The feeling mode included non-logical yes-no decisions and the emotions. The sensations were those of sight, touch, hearing, smell and taste (I only know what I can see). The intuitive mode included all that

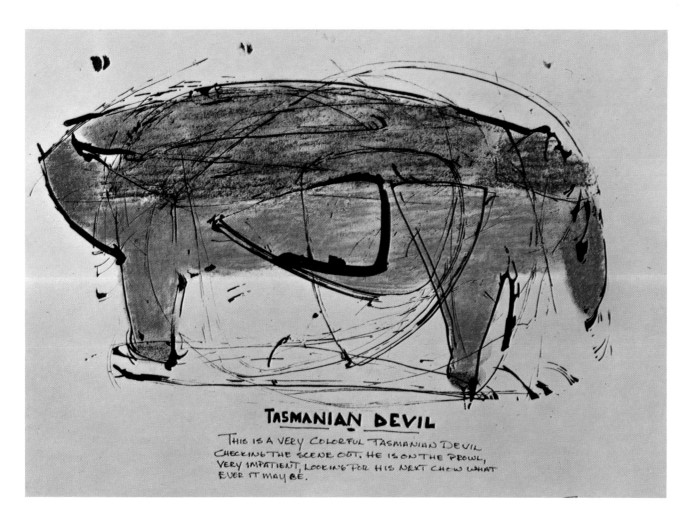

TASMANIAN DEVIL

THIS IS A VERY COLORFUL TASMANIAN DEVIL CHECKING THE SCENE OUT. HE IS ON THE PROWL, VERY IMPATIENT, LOOKING FOR HIS NEXT CHOW WHAT EVER IT MAY BE.

TED'S Devil may be conflicted about some issues, judging from the two heads on his colorful body.

knowledge which is inherent in the race — our "genetic" knowledge, appreciation of aesthetics, and the capacity for conceiving possibilities for things not yet visible in both the outer world and the spiritual realm.

Jung suggested that we usually develop one or two of these psychological functions, which he called superior, and neglected one or two, to which he referred as inferior. He felt that people could look at themselves and note which functions they had neglected, develop these more fully, and as a consequence, enjoy life more fully.

Currently, the Western world is predominantly "left-hemisphere" oriented, and as a consequence, the irrational, intuitive qualities of the right brain which help make people creative have not been fully valued and developed . . . hence the false premise exists that art is a frill, and therefore it is not fully integrated as an essential part of our educational system.

Another concept of art therapy is that all the marks we make on paper, all the colors and graphic gestures we choose and use are extensions of ourselves and what we are thinking and feeling. Therefore, any drawing can be used as a projective technique, by having people draw, and then describe what they see in the drawing they have done. The assumption is that whatever they say about their drawings is in a very real sense a description of how they perceive themselves and the world.

These drawings may be either directed or spontaneous. In directed drawings, people are asked to draw pictures of people, houses, their families, animals or fantasies in their minds' eyes. Spontaneous drawings may be abstract or representational. In either case, when describing what they have drawn, they are elucidating their own dynamics. This process may be facilitated by the gestalt technique of having them describe themselves in the first person singular, as the object they have drawn.

INTERPRETATION

It is unnecessary for anyone to assume the role of interpreter, and tell the artists what their drawings mean. Such interpretation tends to close off the communication process; it can leave the artists who have become vulnerable by self-disclosure feeling invaded by an authority telling them what,

19

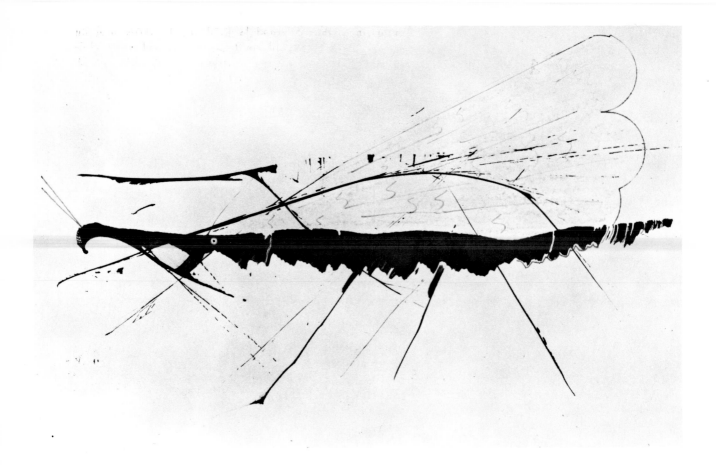

DICK, a young black TV actor, writes:

"This is an afid. He is tired
of being considered an insect, so
he now becomes larger than life
to show his true beauty."

how and who they really are. Open-ended questions (i.e. questions that can't be answered by a "yes" or "no") can be asked to to allow for greater comprehension, but interpretations often tend to destroy the comfortable and safe environment necessary for openness, insight and growth.

Both directed and spontaneous drawing techniques have their own special values. However, when people are allowed to draw freely, their anxieties about their "products" are lessened, allowing for freer expression and creativity.

Another concept of art therapy is that art allows working through conflicts on paper, with clay and with other media. Anger, guilt, fear and other subliminal emotions may not only be expressed graphically, but while being explored in a series of drawings or sculptures, these feelings may at the same time be resolved and/or integrated; sequestered energies may be released and destructive impulses channeled, and all without the use of words.

This aspect is what makes art therapy valuable as an adjunct to verbal therapy; and especially valuable, therefore, for those for whom words are too easy or too hard. But it is, above all, a mode of education of those functions which are best reached non-verbally.

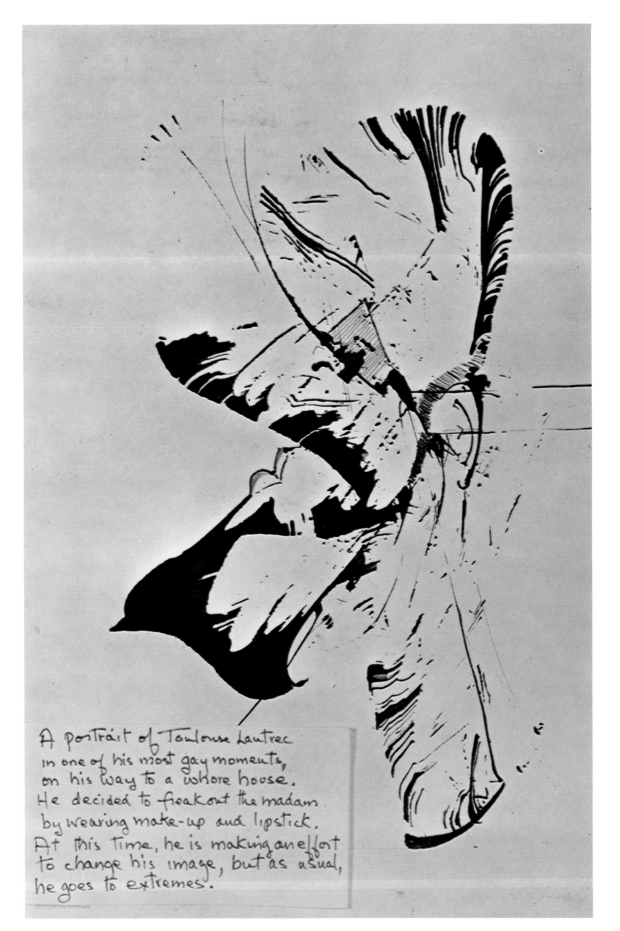

A portrait of Toulouse Lautrec
in one of his most gay moments,
on his way to a whore house.
He decided to freak out the madam
by wearing make-up and lipstick.
At this time, he is making an effort
to change his image, but as usual,
he goes to extremes.

21

DICK, too, may be unconsciously dealing
with some strong conflicts about his
sexual identity.

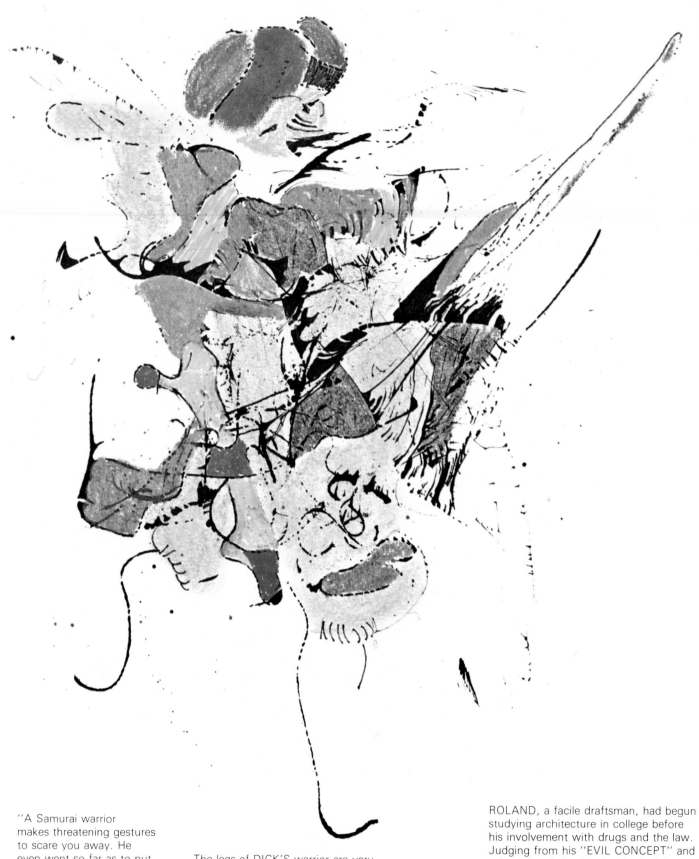

22

"A Samurai warrior
makes threatening gestures
to scare you away. He
even went so far as to put
fake blood on his blade;
but really, he is a sensitive
and passive warrior.

He must keep his guard up
and his colorful show going."

The legs of DICK'S warrior are very
flimsy, substantiating his feelings
of fear and inadequacy.

Dick is now pursuing a colorful
career on TV; I hope he has let
his guard down a little.

ROLAND, a facile draftsman, had begun
studying architecture in college before
his involvement with drugs and the law.
Judging from his "EVIL CONCEPT" and
subsequent behavior, he clearly felt
that he had no control over his behavior.
He left the rehabilitation program with
a great deal of money belonging to
his fellow patients. Currently, he has
dropped out of sight.

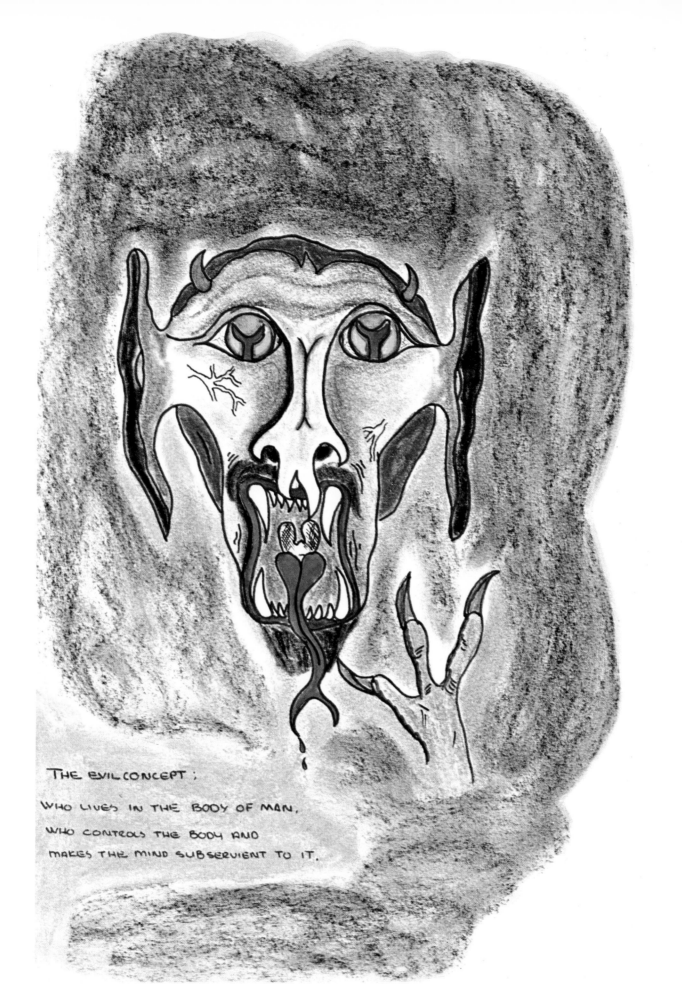

THE EVIL CONCEPT:

WHO LIVES IN THE BODY OF MAN,
WHO CONTROLS THE BODY AND
MAKES THE MIND SUBSERVIENT TO IT.

23

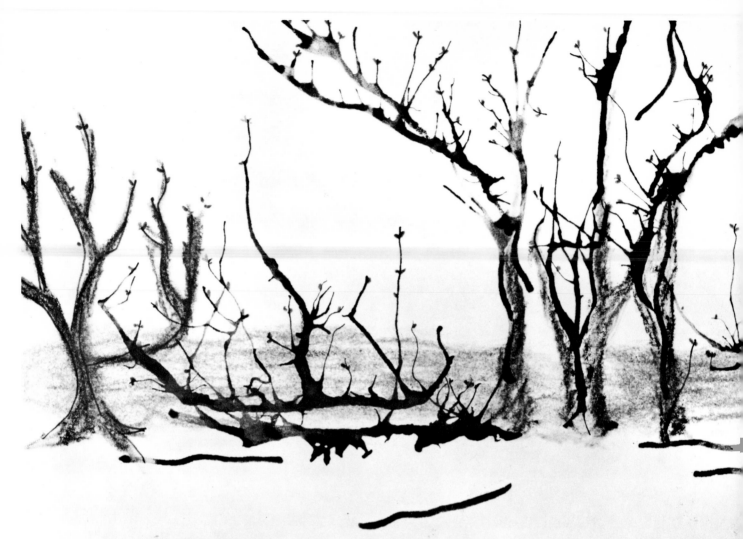

THE FOREST

THE FOREST AFTER A FIRE, THAT BROUGHT DESTRUCTION AND RUIN:
AFTER A TIME THE FORCE THAT FOREST HOLDS ON TO BRINGS NEW LIFE:
STRUGELING TO PUT FORTH NEW LIFE, THE FOREST PUSHES FORWARD,
SOMETHINGS WILL CHANGE BECAUSE OF THE RUIN, BUT NEW BRANCHES
REPLACE THE OLD. THE CHANGE COMES ABOUT SLOW BUT SURE:
MY LIFE IS THAT FOREST, TIRED BEAT AND IN RUIN. THE PROMISE
TO US ALL IS THAT THE FOREST WILL GROW AGAIN AND YOUR LIFE
WILL BE NEW AGAIN. WITH GREEN AND COOL STREAMS' PASSING THROUGH

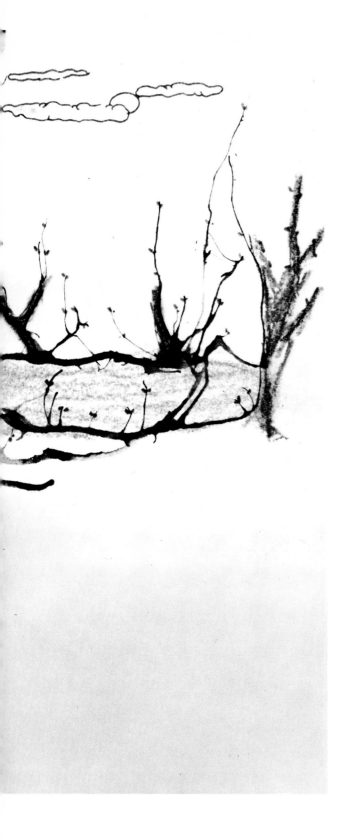

ROLAND'S landscape is indeed barren.
His trees show a little hope with
their tiny green shoots appearing,
but the way he changes his pronouns
"my life" to "your life" in mid-
paragraph would seem to indicate that
he doesn't really believe that his life
will be new again.

25

J., in the detoxification program at the hospital, has spent many of his fifty years in prison. In a small drawing he did on the reverse side of the page, is a seated figure by a barred window, holding his bowed head in his hands. He saw no relationship between his drawings and his life, probably because of the lack of pupil in his "polluted eye".

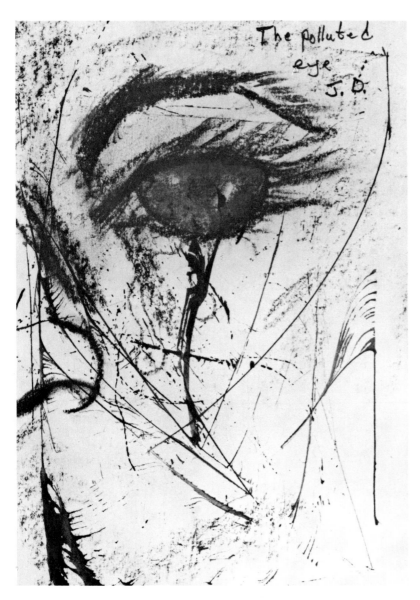

The polluted eye J. D.

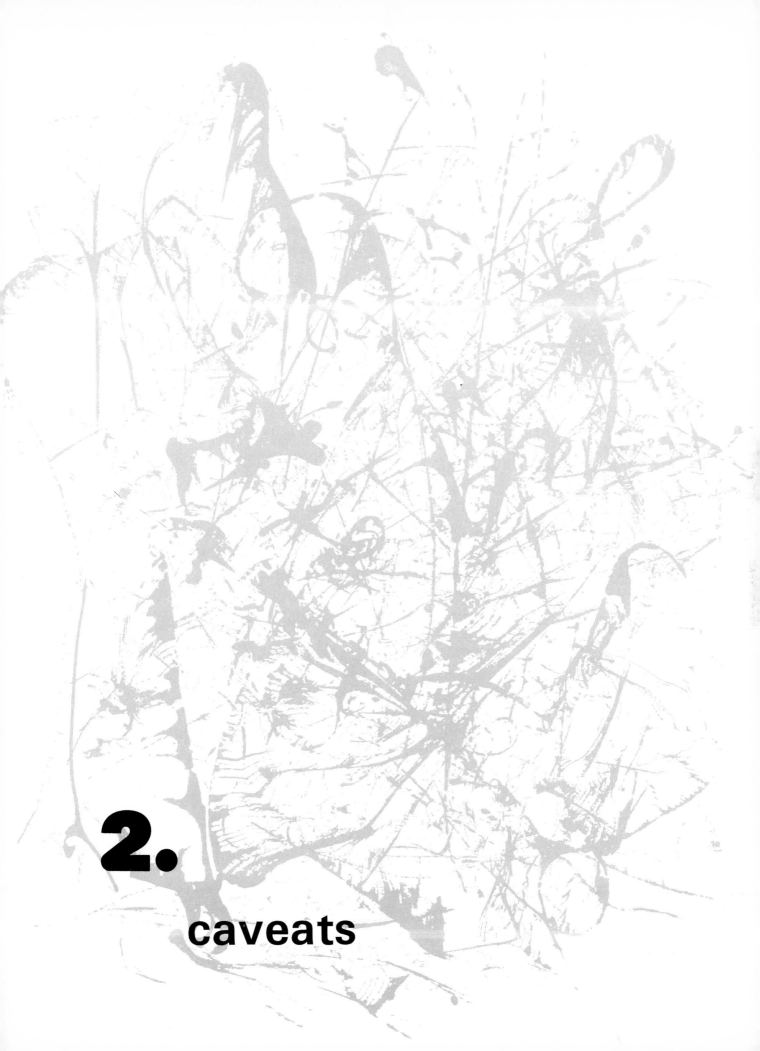

2.

caveats

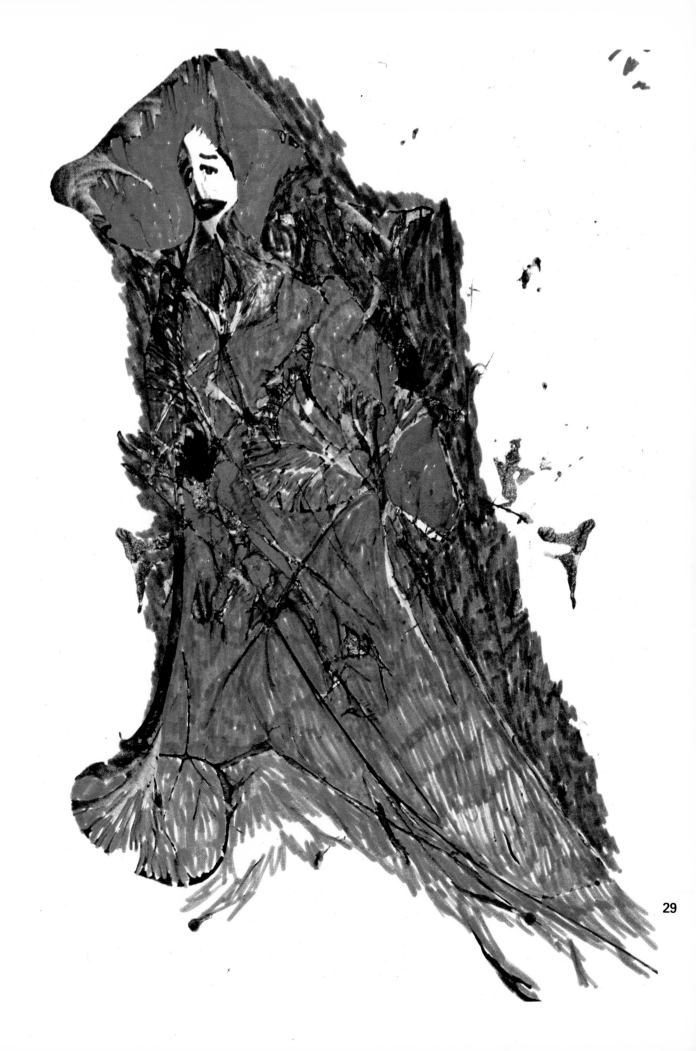

29

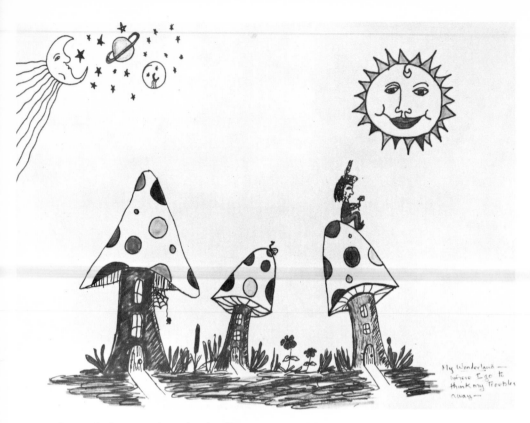

Using all the shades of red and orange she could find, LISA covered the paper. She had given herself permission to express herself more openly. She found a face hiding behind her intense colors, and she wrote: "A scared person hiding behind her anger. Angry at the world, angry at herself. Will she come out of this anger or keep hiding behind it?"

LISA died of an overdose shortly after she quit the program, leaving a small baby. She had never in her 20 years worked at any steady employment. Her first drawing in the Art Therapy program said: "My Wonderland, where I go to think my troubles away."

She was distrustful of everyone and was not about to reveal anything emotional in her work.

As the role of art therapy has grown in the helping professions within the past twenty years, it has become clear that many aspects of the art therapy process have universal significance.

The word "therapy" however, gives a medical connotation to art therapy implying that one would have to be "ill" to need art therapy. For me, and for many other humanistically-oriented art therapists, this is simply not true. Art therapy does not have to be reserved for those who are emotionally disturbed or "mentally ill", or for those who are out of the mainstream of our culture. It is indeed valuable for those people, but the techniques of art therapy developed while working with them has also proved useful for the "normal and well adjusted", and can improve the quality of life for all of us.

In the acquisition of social skills, we all strike a balance for ourselves between inhibition and expression of feelings. Unfortunately, most of us learn inhibition somewhat better than expression; it is safer. Art therapy can provide a place and method for experimentation with the expression of feelings that can be safe, revelatory, fulfilling, and generally satisfying. Some such experience may be necessary for emotional development and growth.

But before I suggest some simple experiences in art which are useful for facilitating the flow of feelings onto paper, I would like to stress two of the basic concepts and cautions of the process of art therapy.

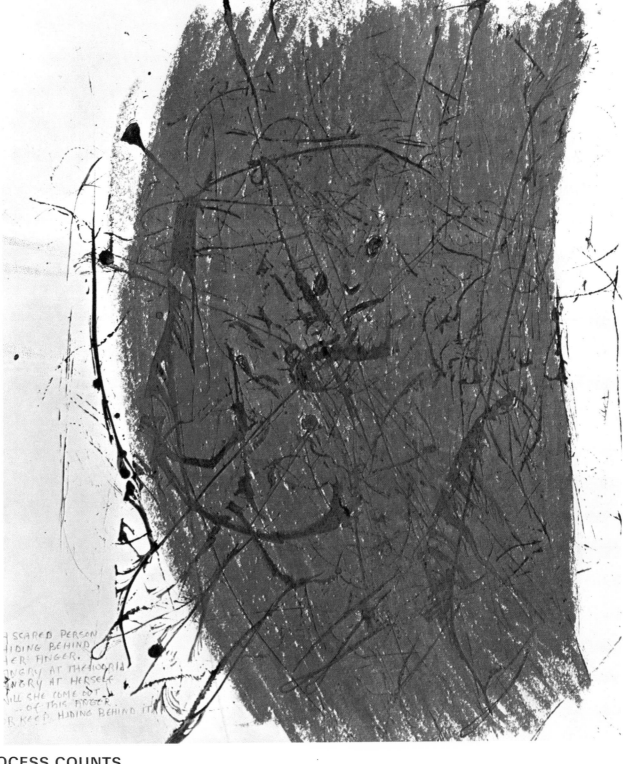

A SCARED PERSON
HIDING BEHIND
HER FINGER.
ANGRY AT THE WORLD
ANGRY AT HERSELF
WILL SHE COME OUT
OF THIS FINGER
OR KEEP HIDING BEHIND IT

HE PROCESS COUNTS

First, if art therapy had a motto, it would be: "IT IS THE PROCESS, NOT THE PRODUCT, THAT COUNTS." The use of art materials, the gestures, the feelings behind them, are the important aspect, how it looks aesthetically to the viewer is not of concern at all. The feeling about the colors and lines; the feelings about space or lack of space, are of concern, not that the perspective may be off, or that the object may not look "right". We have learned, (and in our society it is important to learn) to measure, compare, judge and evaluate.

This critical faculty we have so thoroughly developed is not, however, compatible with the art therapy process; it effectively cuts off the flow and expression of imagery. Someone who is asked to draw how they feel, and then is measured by the yardstick of aesthetics, will feel betrayed, and will repress further feelings. Creativity of expression is stifled by judgmental evaluation.

Is it not important to learn good from bad art? Not when one is involved in the art therapy process. The expression of feelings at this time has

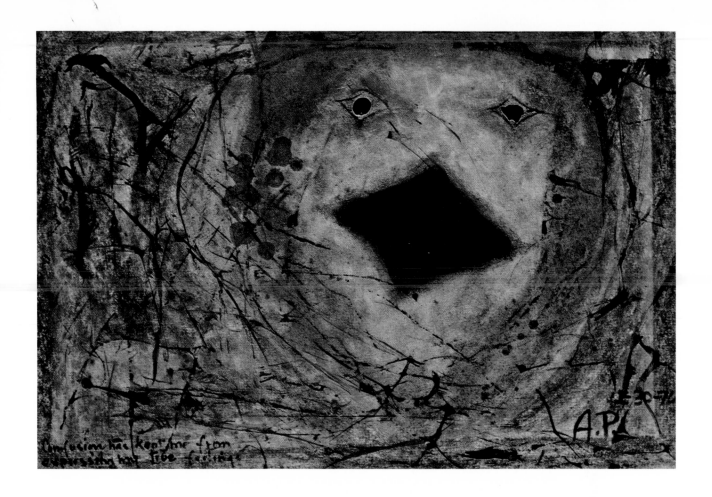

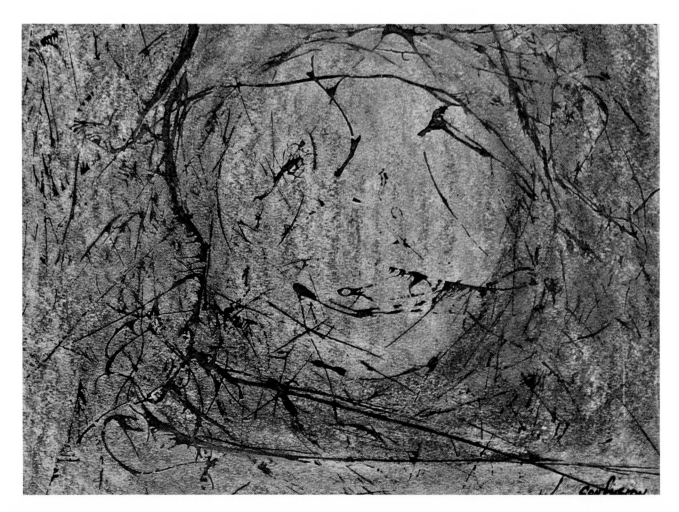

HARRY, a 35 year old car salesman and
house painter, said he got into drugs
at age 20 to "follow the crowd".

When I asked him what the mouth was
trying to say, he replied that he was
not about to talk about what was going
on inside because once he started,
he might not be able to stop....and
he might reveal some "terrible" things.
He wrote: "Listening in confusion."

Two weeks later, HARRY returned to
Art Therapy, and drew the lower drawing.
It is a colorless version of the one
above, confirming that he was not about
to reveal his fears and his "terrible
thoughts". He had not recalled his
previous drawing, but his artwork showed
he had not forgotten his resolve.

He later sculpted a small bust of a man with
no eyes or ears, and a firmly set mouth,
and left the rehabilitation program
soon after, taking his secrets with him.

nothing to do with learning art, per se. I do believe
however, that after one has learned to use art
materials to express feelings, the motivation to
accept the discipline of art will follow closely.

FEELINGS AND EMOTIONS

The second concept is of equal importance.
Artwork may evoke some feelings in the viewer,
but these feelings are not necessarily the emotions
the artist was trying to express. If the viewer is not
aware that frequently the two sets of feelings can
be quite different, he may assume, incorrectly, that
the artist is feeling the same way. In addition, projection often attributes to other persons those
objectionable characteristics which one wishes to
disclaim in oneself. In art therapy, projection can
be useful or destructive.

I feel that a good way to resolve this is to ASK
the artist what the picture means. Do not tell, do
not interpret; and also, do not even require an
answer. This is really necessary, in order to provide
a safe environment where people can feel comfortable and accepted while expressing themselves
on paper, or in other media, any way they can, or
wish. Telling is often projection; interpretation is
tricky and difficult, even for professional therapists; non-professionals, no matter how confident
or full of good will, should leave both strictly alone.
Both telling and interpretation can close off the
expression of feeling by the time you are halfway
through the first sentence. Also, people are often
not immediately aware of the emotional significance of their drawings, or they may not be "ready"
to deal with it. Like dreams, the act of drawing
brings subliminal thoughts and feelings closer to
the conscious mind. If there is a hint of coercion,
of demand to share meanings, the phantom neb-
ulous feelings may submerge, and the artist may
retreat into stereotypical artwork.

With these caveats in mind, I will discuss in the
next chapter some exercises which are appropriate
for "normal" people of any age, by themselves,
following the simple directions, and without the
need for the art therapist's expertise.

"MONKEY SEE, MONKEY WONDER —
This monkey is checking things out —
Monkey sits and climbs up high to
stay out of the way of the elephant."

She could see that she did feel that
part of her was passive and watchful,
but that there was a strong and powerful
part of her represented by the elephant.

MINDY completed the rehabilitation
program and is now working with drug
addicts. She wrote: "Deepness — The
weirdness and freak in people that is
always covered up." She, too, struggled
to be open and honest with her feelings,
more successfully than did HARRY.

34

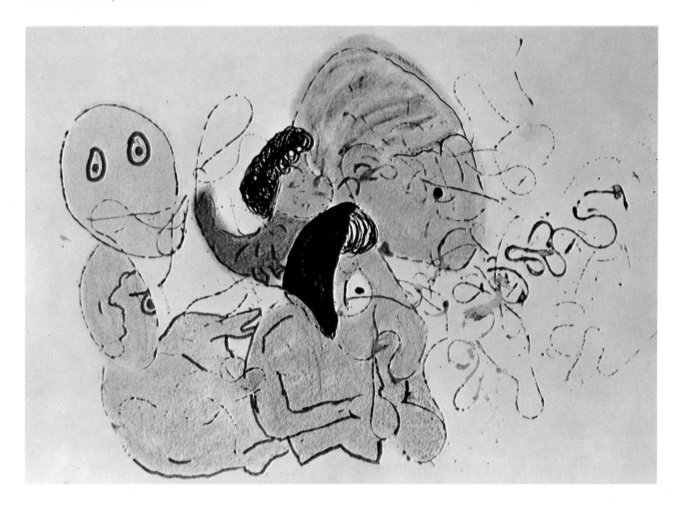

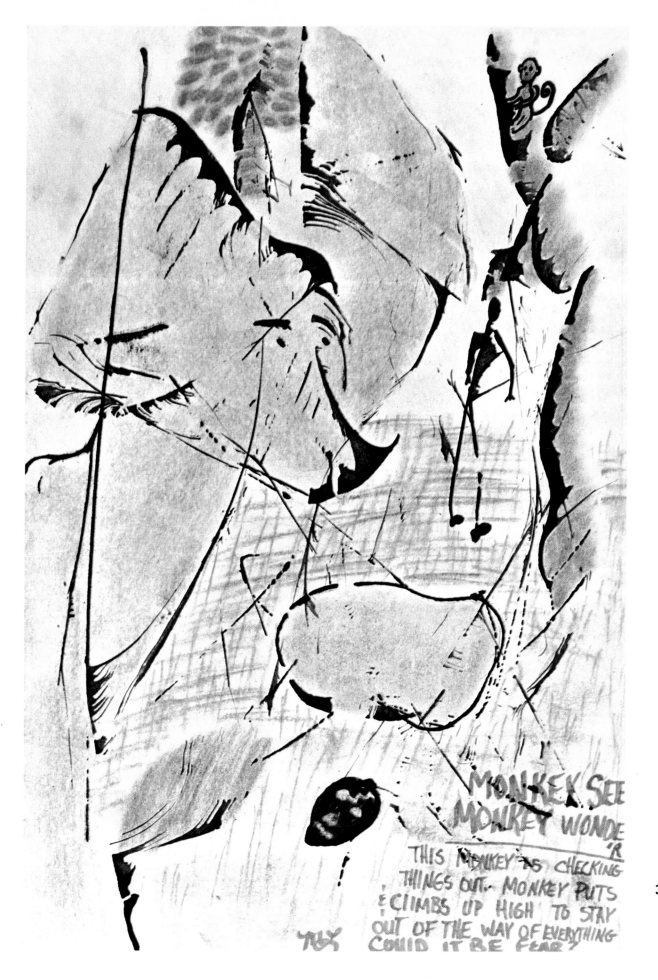

MONKEY SEE
MONKEY WONDER

THIS MONKEY IS CHECKING
THINGS OUT. MONKEY PUTS
& CLIMBS UP HIGH TO STAY
OUT OF THE WAY OF EVERYTHING
COULD IT BE FEAR?

35

"This is Herkimer Snerd
Did you hear what he heard?
He thinks its quite absurd,
But doesn't say a word."

Many times when people draw hats, they are saying they don't want to talk about their feelings. This was certainly the case with Kathleen.

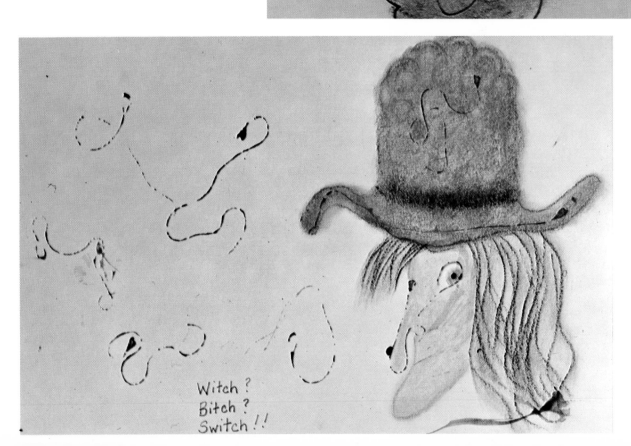

Witch ?
Bitch ?
Switch !!

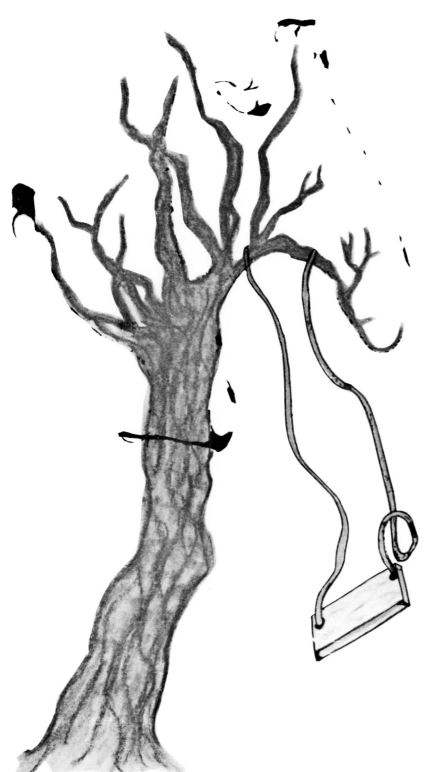

KATHLEEN was very resistant to art therapy.
She worked for 3 hours on each of her
drawings, and reluctantly wrote on
some of them.

Her last drawing, the tree with the looped
swing, does not augur well for her, as loops sometimes
foretell an unconscious self-destructiveness. I have
lost track of KATHLEEN.

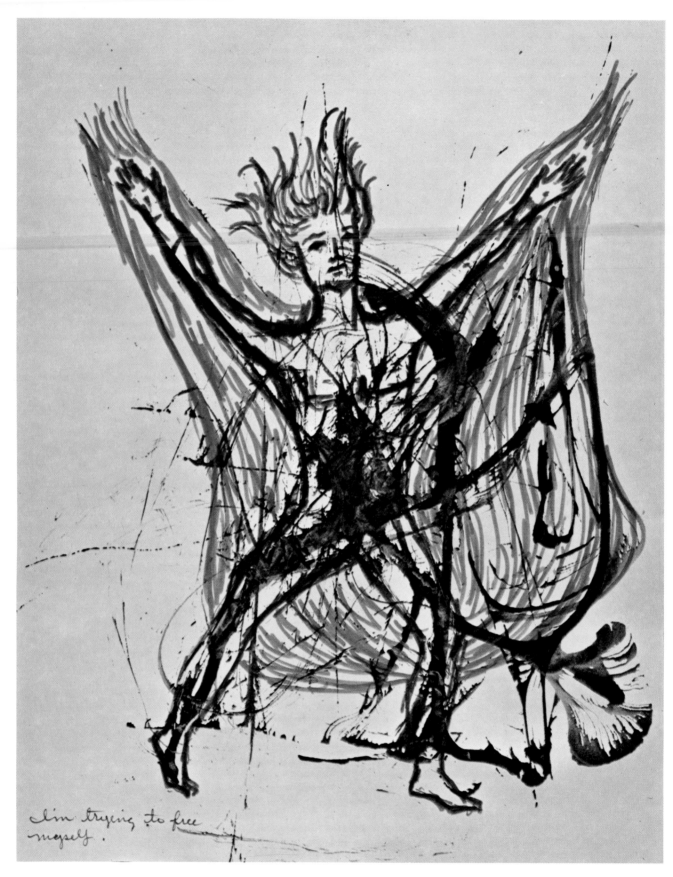

I'm trying to free myself.

38

PHIL, a hairdresser, drew
a powerful cape of color around himself,
as if he were on fire,
as he wrote: "I'm trying to free myself."

WAYNE, in and out of prison for many of his 25 years, states his perception of himself: "A Bull that fights for his life because it's the only way he knows."

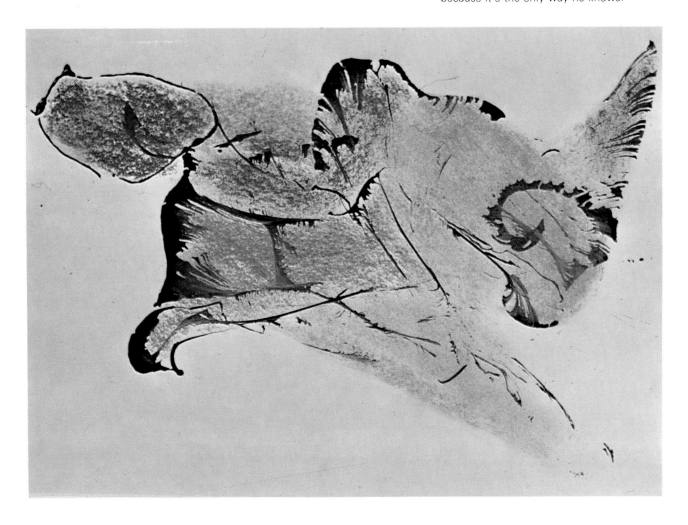

39

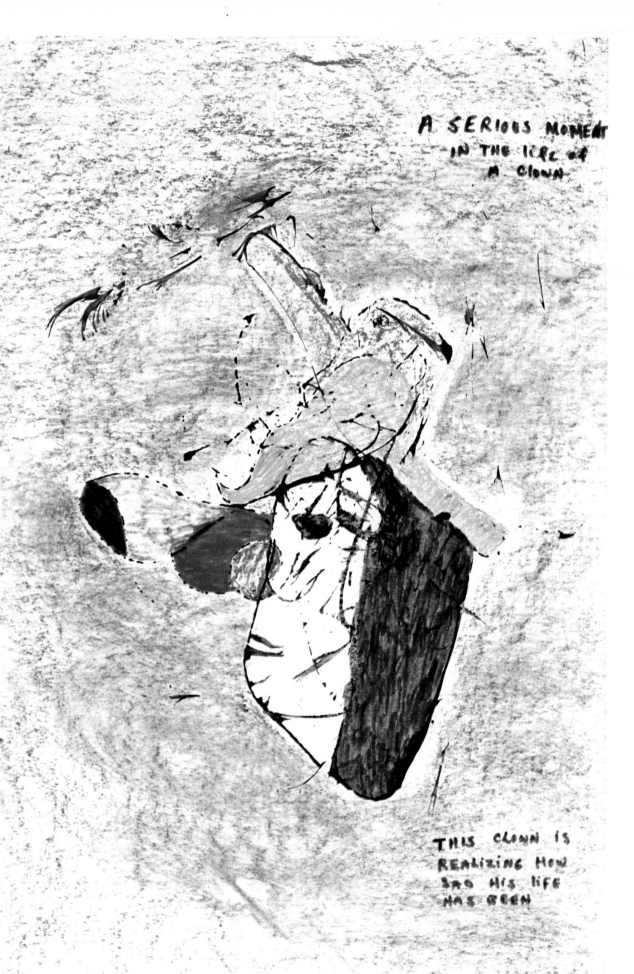

A SERIOUS MOMENT
IN THE LIFE OF
A CLOWN

THIS CLOWN IS
REALIZING HOW
SAD HIS LIFE
HAS BEEN

40

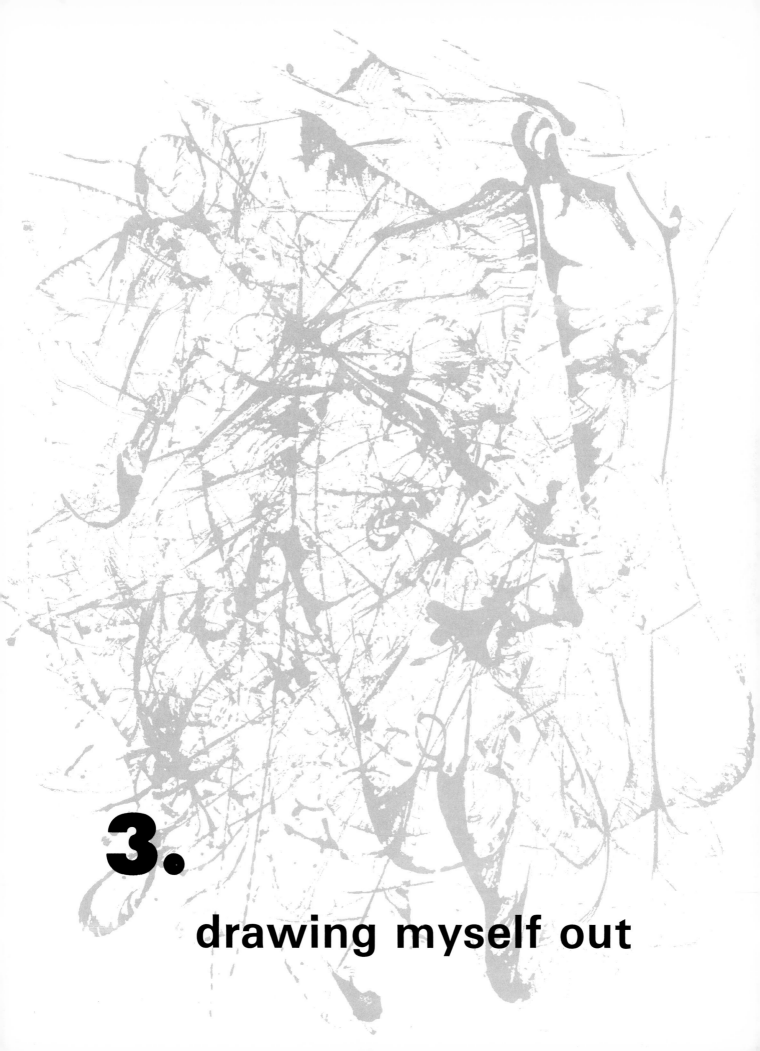

3.
drawing myself out

MIKE enjoyed working with the art materials and frequently chose to make no statement. His butterfly was the only part of the drawing he did not plan. It just happened.

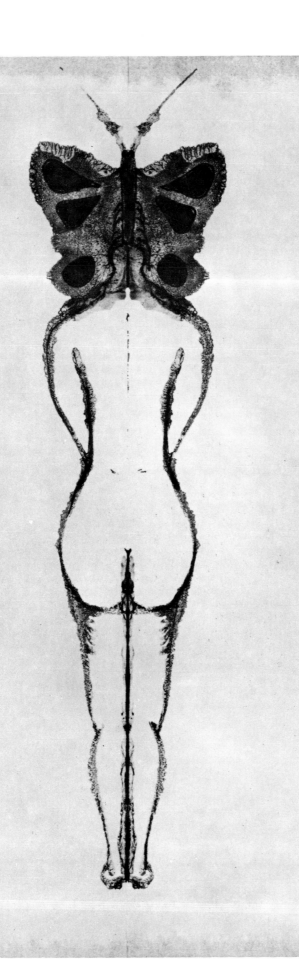

43

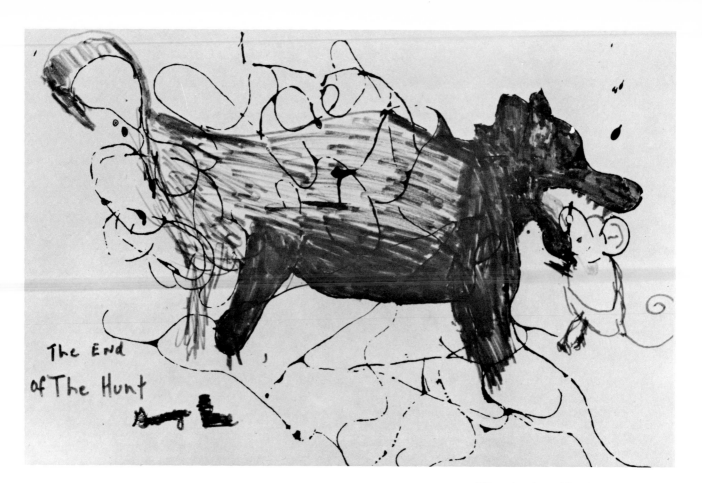

The End
of The Hunt

A s I said, every mark we make on paper, all the colors and graphic gestures and forms we create are extensions of ourselves, how we are thinking and feeling, and how we see the world. I think that you may become more fully aware of this if you do the following two exercises.

You will need paper (11x16 will do), and a selection of felt-tipped pens, pastels and crayons, and have the materials easy to reach. You may do this by yourself, or in a group.

Now what kind of marks are we talking about?

Let us create two animals on one piece of paper. These are going to be fantasy animals, so that you can make up your own animals, or you can borrow from different ones in your own combinations. Remember that they don't have to look like anything you've ever seen before. And they are not going to be "graded." You can use any of the drawing materials you wish. Take about ten minutes for the drawing. Don't read further until you have done the drawing.

Now, describe the animals you have drawn. Write down three adjectives about them on the paper. Note what expressions the animals have. Are you able to make up something the animals might want to say to each other? Can you write free verse or a fantasy about what the animals might say and do?

POLARITIES

As you may have experienced when you drew the two animals, the second animal often has contrasting qualities from the first. This exercise generally will reveal polarities, contrasts or conflicts within a person; it will show different, sometimes opposing facets of personality. This is normal. In addition, you can be aware of whether the animals are whole or parts; very often the parts which are left out may be of significance for the artist. For example, the absence of a mouth may suggest difficulty in communicating; the absence of hands or feet, helplessness. If the animals are facing away from each other, it is possible that they have a conflict which is difficult to resolve. Are the animals standing on the ground? If not, they may have a feeling of insecurity. The relative size of the animals to each other and to the paper may give a clue to their feelings of importance.

As you describe your animals, it should in time become rather obvious that you are describing qualities that you may have yourself. If this makes you very uncomfortable, you may be overly critical of yourself. It is rather common for people to feel embarassed about how they see themselves, and afraid of revealing these very private things. If you can adopt a gentle and accepting attitude toward yourself, you will see that you are, even as we and they, human. If in addition, you can share these things, in a supportive group, you will find comfort

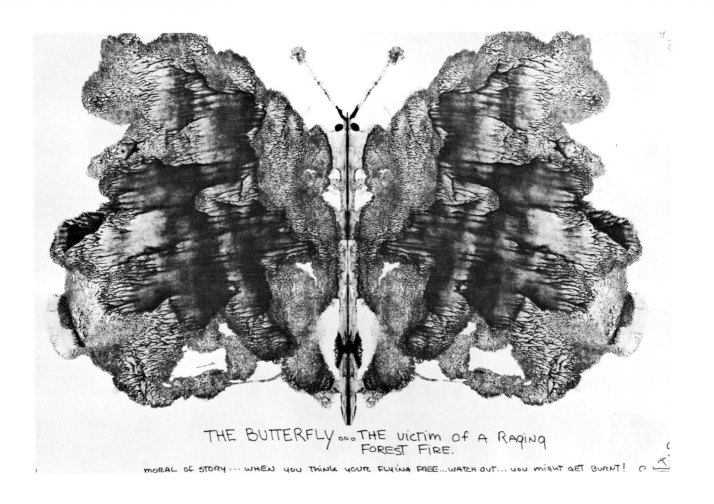

THE BUTTERFLY...THE VICTIM OF A RAGING
FOREST FIRE.

MORAL OF STORY...WHEN YOU THINK YOU'RE FLYING FREE...WATCH OUT...YOU MIGHT GET BURNT!

MIKE's butterfly reappeared, with more of a story — "The Butterfly — The victim of a Raging Forest Fire." Apparently MIKE felt helpless about his addiction, a victim of fate.

in knowing that others in the group may not only not be shocked or critical, but accepting and forgiving; they probably have the same critical internal voices, too, and the experience of sharing can draw people closer. You may be surprised to find how universal are feelings and characteristics you thought unique to you.

For the second exercise, you will need a method for creating a meaningless group of marks on paper. I generally use string dipped in ink or diluted poster paint, dragged across the paper, for a minute or two, as was done with many of the drug addicts' drawings.

Then turn the paper around, sideways and upside down until you discover an image or several images you wish to develop further with the other art materials, bringing what you see into better focus. Allow about ten minutes for this activity. Now write a fantasy, free verse or title about your creation. You might imagine being what you have created as Fritz Perls has suggested in Gestalt Therapy, and write a story about what you would do and feel as this creation.

If you are in a group, observe for yourself the variety of images. Is your image fragmented?....are there several small disjointed images on one page? Possibly you were anxious and confused, and had a difficult time focusing, this time.

45

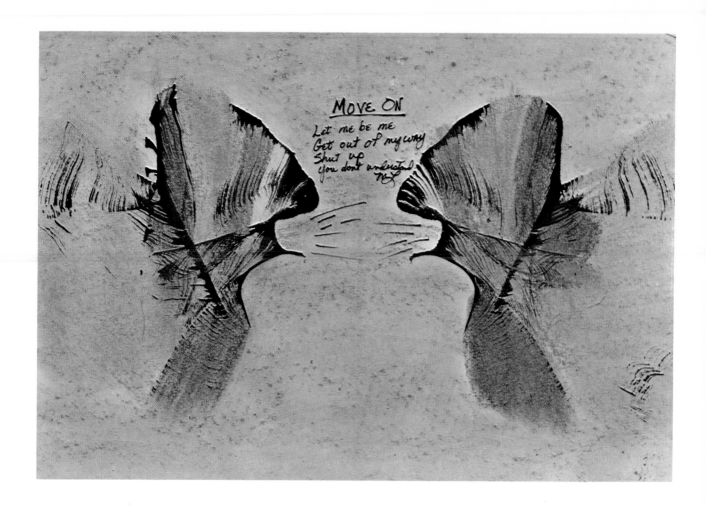

MINDY allowed her mirror images to imitate life and her internal bickering voices.

THE METAPHOR OF ART

Is the image rigid? Are you feeling tight and controlled? The use of soft pastels and paints can help you relax and let the feelings flow.

Is the image uncontained and formless? Sometimes, just limiting yourself to felt-tipped pens and other easily controlled materials can help eliminate confusion and establish feelings of control in both art and behavior.

Is the image frightening or frightened? Sometimes people feeling overwhelmed by the world find it easier to deal with and express their anxiety nonverbally.

Are there drawings which use no color, although color was available? Sometimes the use of color can be threatening, because it can release emotions the person doesn't want to feel or deal with.

Is the drawing a blaze of color? Many people feel more comfortable using color on paper than expressing their emotions verbally.

Pay attention if possible to how you have put your colors down....in what order, and perhaps in layers. Sometimes a cool color covering a warm color might be saying "hide that feeling."

46

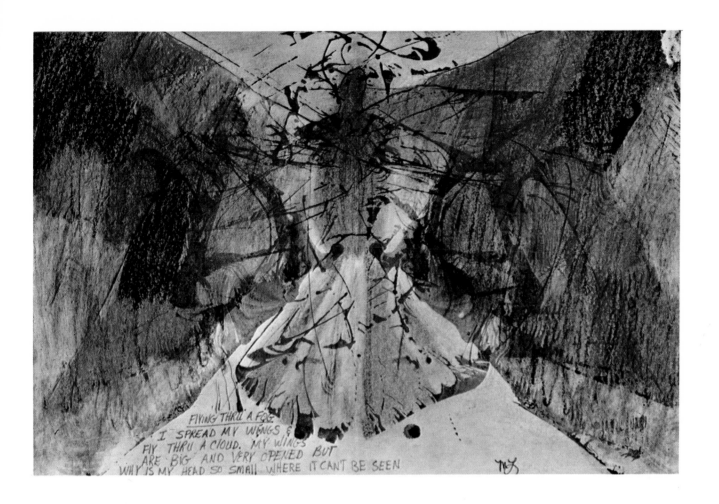

FLYING THRU A FOG
I SPREAD MY WINGS &
FLY THRU A CLOUD. MY WINGS
ARE BIG AND VERY OPENED BUT
WHY IS MY HEAD SO SMALL WHERE IT CAN'T BE SEEN

There are endless possibilities. I must stress that they may remain only possibilities. It is a paradox that probing can easily cut off the flow of images. Too bright a light is frightening. It is sufficient to create an environment where people will produce the images without having to talk about them. Many will be willing to share openly, others will not, and their wishes to participate at their own speed should be respected.

If you can create an environment where the right brain processes can be allowed to function, this itself is tremendously helpful and therapeutic. As time goes on, awareness will come, self-images change and conflicts resolve themselves, even without words, using the language of art.

Most of the patients had no feelings
of self worth. They felt that they
had no control over their behavior and
they were helpless, frightened and
frightening, even to themselves.

WILLIAM finally, after much encouragement,
wrote on his folded inkblot, "This is a
unordinary creature reaching out to others."
After this drawing, it was easier for him to
start expressing his feelings and making
friends.

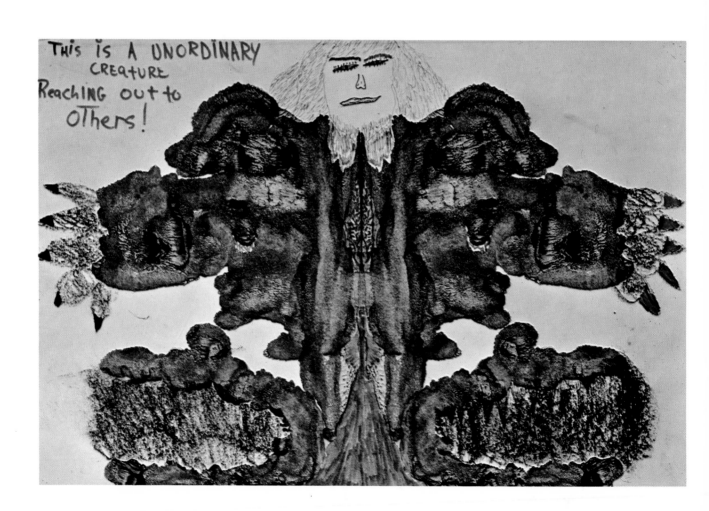

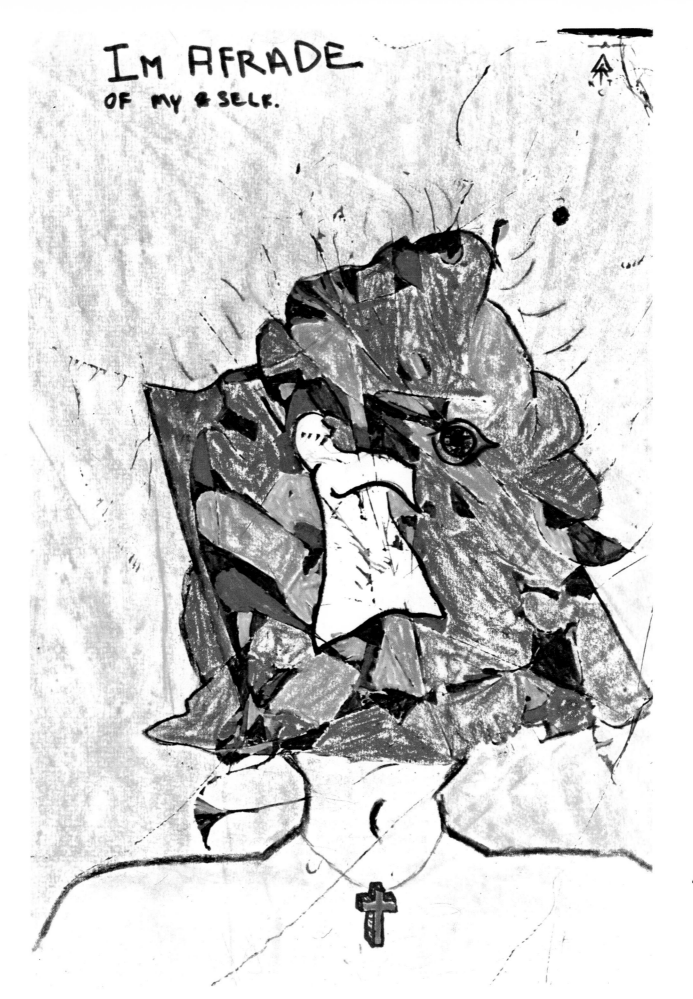

IM AFRADE
OF MY @ SELF.

49

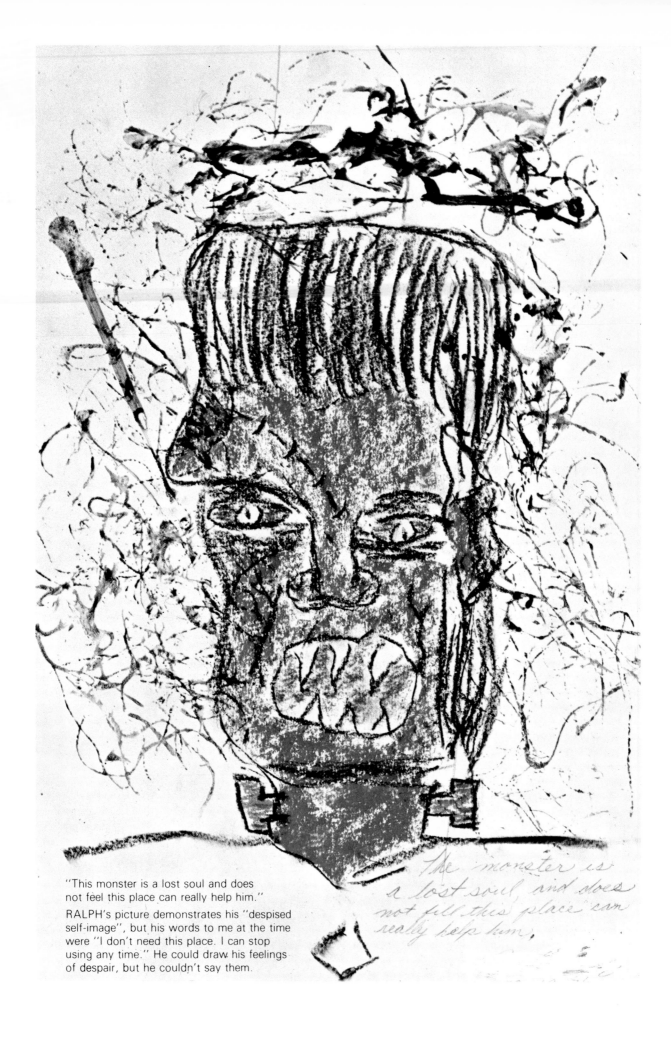

"This monster is a lost soul and does not feel this place can really help him."

RALPH's picture demonstrates his "despised self-image", but his words to me at the time were "I don't need this place. I can stop using any time." He could draw his feelings of despair, but he couldn't say them.

50

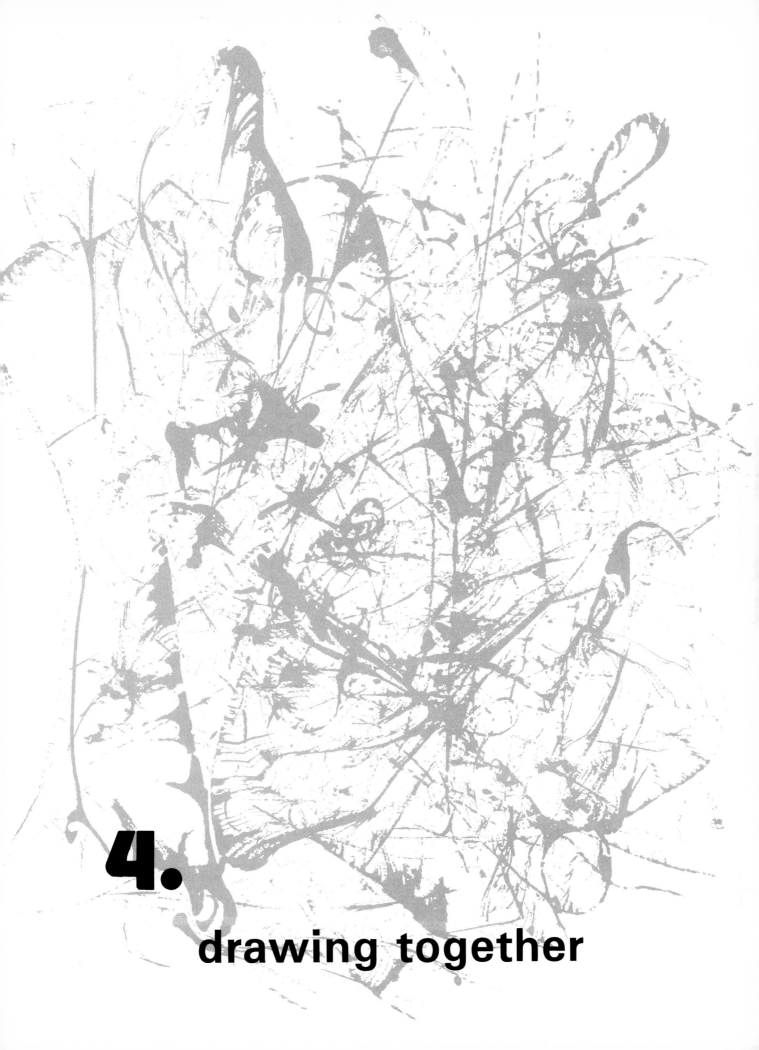

4.
drawing together

Artists have always known that there has been more dimension to people than the rational man would have us believe, but these qualities have been but dimly understood. New physiological and experimental information has shed some additional light which may make it easier for us to understand more parts of ourselves, and to express more of these parts, graphically in art, poetry, dance and music, and to understand these expressions in others.

Joseph Bogen, a neurosurgeon, and Roger Sperry, a neurobiologist, described severe epileptic patients who required an operation in which the corpus callosum, which connects the two hemispheres of the brain, was severed. When Sperry and Bogen studied them after the two lobes were disconnected, they were able to identify qualities and skills which were then specifically performed by each of the two lobes individually. We, as whole-brained people, integrate the two hemispheres, and they work in a complementary manner. But we now know that these two physiological entities have unique and distinct characteristics which affect our behavior.

In studying these patients, it was found that the left hemisphere appeared to be the logical, verbal part of the brain. It analyzes and processes information in a rational, linear, sequential way.

The right hemisphere is intuitive, able to abstract, wordless and imaginative. It processes our orientation in space, it recognizes forms, and works relationally, acoustically, simultaneously, and more holistically than does the left hemisphere.

How do these concepts relate to fine artists and their art?

It is possible for each of us to become aware of a dominant mode of being and how we express it in our lives. We can also be aware, when we look at artists' work, of which mode was dominant for the artist; their general way of seeing the world would be clearly visible in their work.

Another concomitant of this is the realization that we are most stirred and excited by artists' work which is in the same dominant mode in which we see the world, and possibly we are very disturbed by work done in the opposite modes.

52

THE
FINE ARTIST AND THE

What is more important may be our willingness to see the world through someone else's eyes. Much acrimony and disparagement could be avoided...."Just purely intellectual — there's no feeling to it".... "There is no order to it!"

Most important, however, is an understanding of our own way of seeing the world, and our capacity for growth. For these modes of seeing the world are merely dominant and not fixed. We can develop our inferior functions through awareness, openness, and willingness to explore.

The intellectual mode interprets, translates and verbalizes. A harmonious interplay, working in successive rhythm, is established with intuitive insight, intellectual interpretation, further insight, its interpretation and so on. Through the right brain function of visual and graphic thinking, feelings and ideas can be expressed with simultaneity and sorted out later in an orderly, linear, sequential fashion.

That these concepts now have important experimental and physiological validation may give some of us permission to stop evaluating ourselves in logical analytic ways and to accept and start developing those nonlogical parts of ourselves, which are truly necessary for the artist and the creative process in all of us. In addition, it gives us permission and ability to view all artists' work for what it is: a valid expression of a significant view of the world. The world is larger than any of us can individually comprehend. But we can try!

When we are taught to value all parts of ourselves and to allow more expression of intuition, sensing and feeling; when we perceive our right brain processes as exciting but mysterious, then we can explore these processes with a mixture of curiosity and joy. We can have options of expanding our awareness and making choices about what we want to say and how to go about saying it, more clearly identifying ourselves through our art as unique, individual, and separate.

RIGHT AND LEFT BRAIN

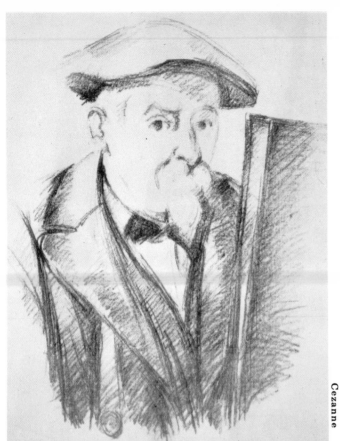

Cezanne

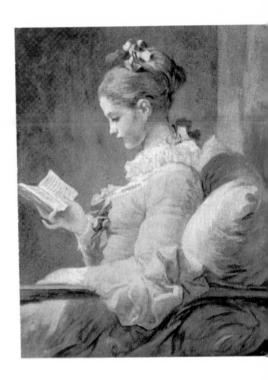

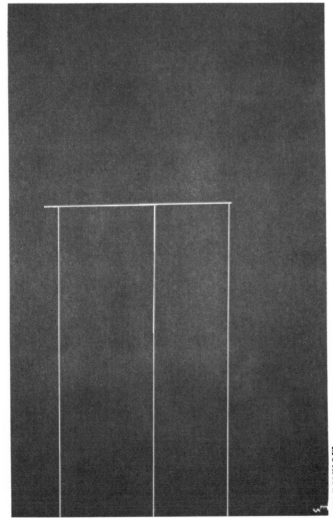

Motherwell

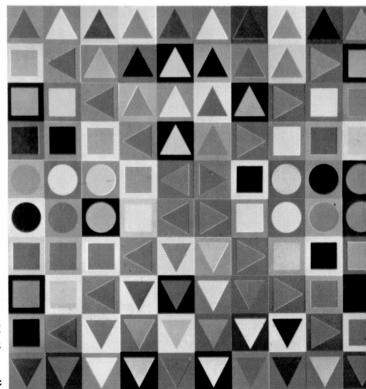

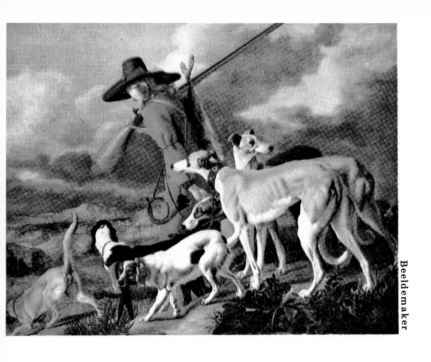

Beeldemaker

HOW YOU SEE YOURSELF AND YOUR WORLD MAY DEPEND ON WHICH SIDE OF THE BRAIN IS DOMINANT FOR YOU. SOCIETY TODAY VALUES AND GEARS EDUCATION TOWARD THE FUNCTIONS OF THE LEFT HEMISPHERE WHICH ARE THE ACTIVE, VERBAL, LOGICAL, SEQUENTIAL AND RATIONAL PARTS OF US.

Some of the many artists who seem to favor the LEFT HEMISPHERE:

Mondrian, Seurat, Pevsner, Albers, Stella, Escher, Warhol, Bridget Riley, Kenneth Noland, Ellsworth Kelly, Robert Irwin, Braque, Lichtenstein, David, Boucher, Watteau.

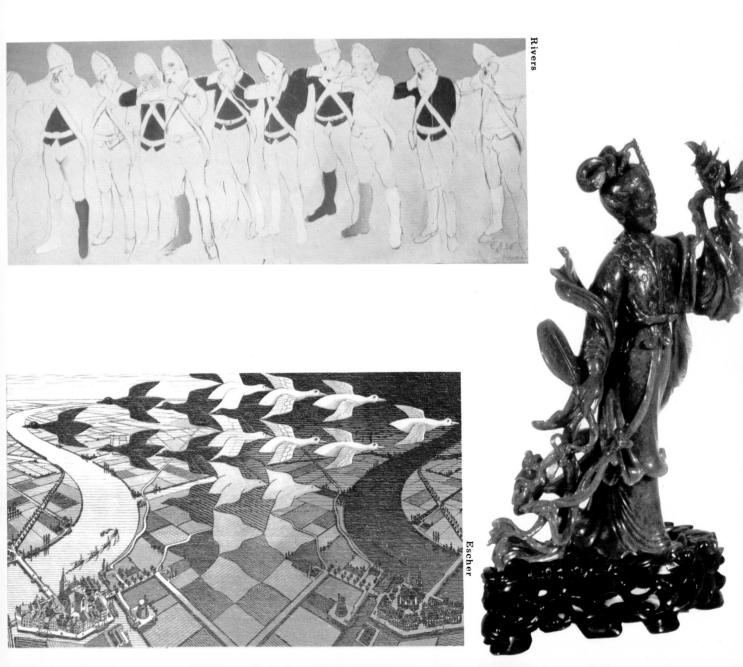

Rivers

Escher

ACTIVE
ANALYTIC
SCIENTIFIC
ORGANIZED
SEQUENTIAL
SHARP FOCUS
INTELLECTUAL
STRUCTURED
LINEAR TIME
CONSCIOUS
RATIONAL
LOGICAL
VERBAL

**LEFT
BRAIN**

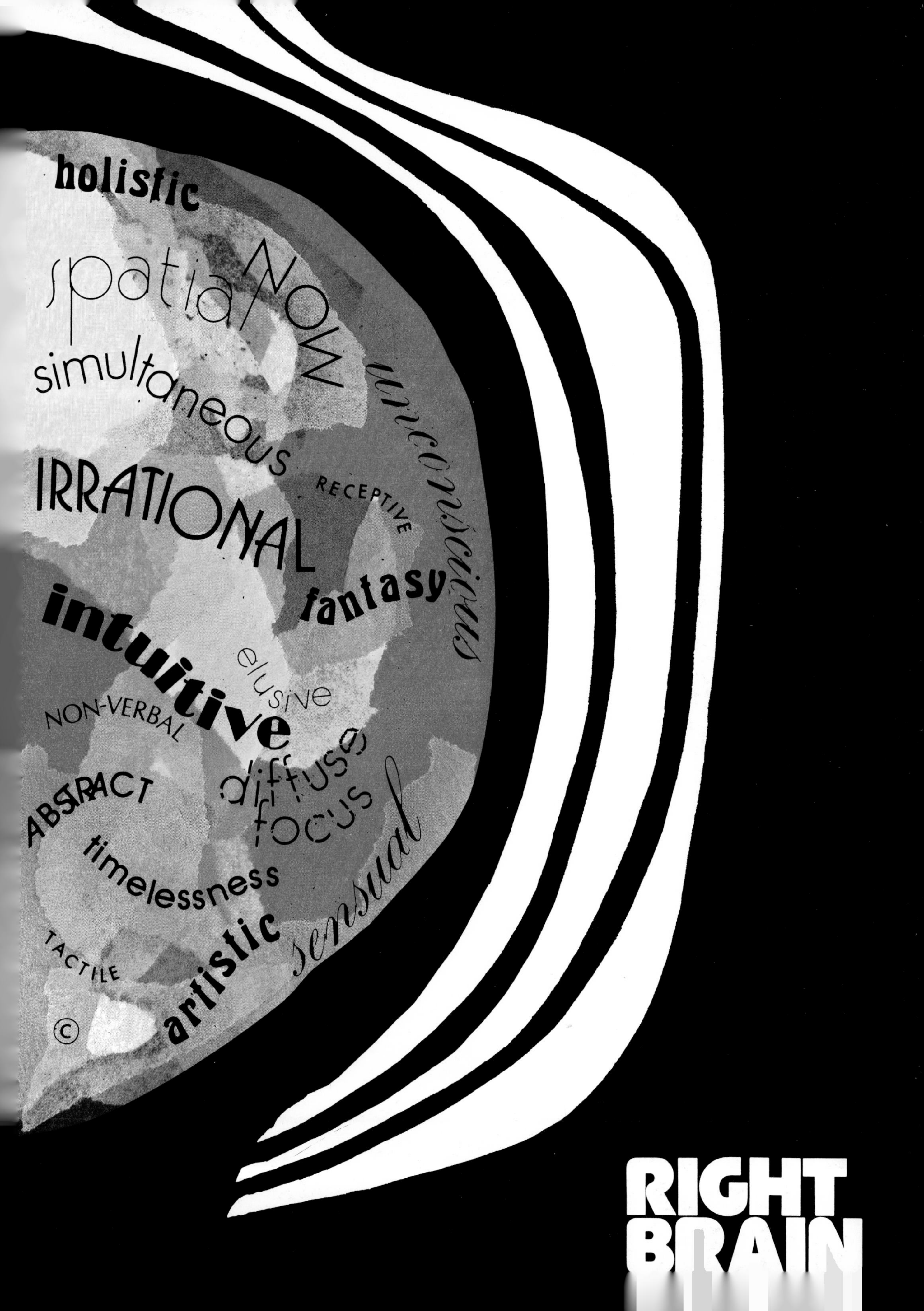

holistic

spatial Now

simultaneous

unconscious

IRRATIONAL

RECEPTIVE

fantasy

intuitive

elusive

NON-VERBAL

diffuse

ABSTRACT

focus

timelessness

sensual

TACTILE

© artistic

RIGHT BRAIN

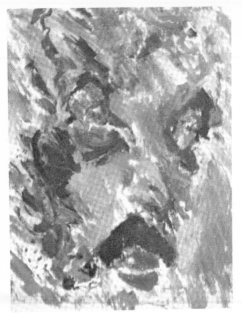

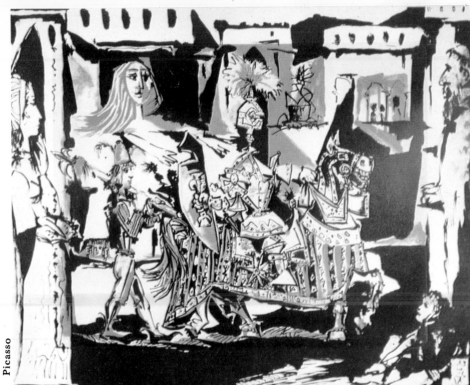

Picasso

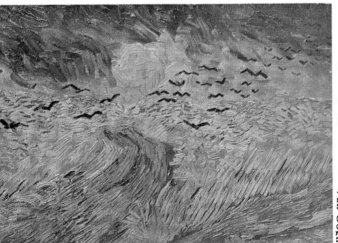

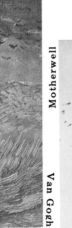

Motherwell

Van Gogh

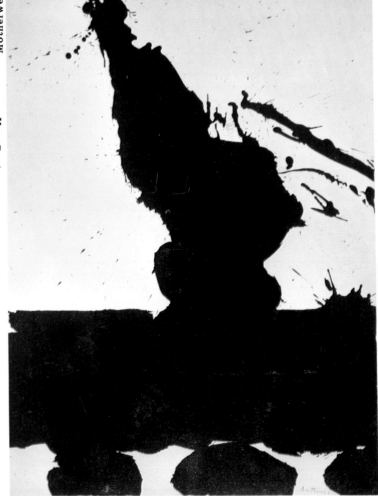

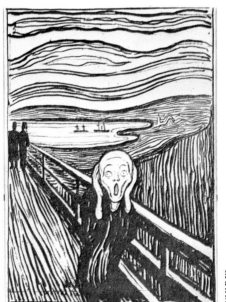

Munch

RIGHT BRAIN

MANY PEOPLE LEARN MORE EFFECTIVELY
THROUGH THEIR RIGHT BRAIN FUNCTIONS.
THESE ARE THE INTUITIVE, NON-VERBAL,
IMAGINATIVE, ELUSIVE PARTS OF ALL OF
US. NO MATTER WHICH HEMISPHERE IS
DOMINANT, WE ALL NEED TO DISCOVER
OUR OWN UNIQUE BALANCE: WE NEED TO USE
BOTH HEMISPHERES IN ORDER TO BE CREATIVE.

Some of the many artists who seem to favor
the RIGHT HEMISPHERE:

Franz Kline, De Kooning, Hans Hoffman, Gorky,
Pollack, Turner, Klee, Frankenthaler, Bosch,
Breugel, Fuseli, Blake, Hunterwasser, Chaqall,
Giacometti, Matisse, Roualt, Van Gogh,
Gauguin, Dubuffet.

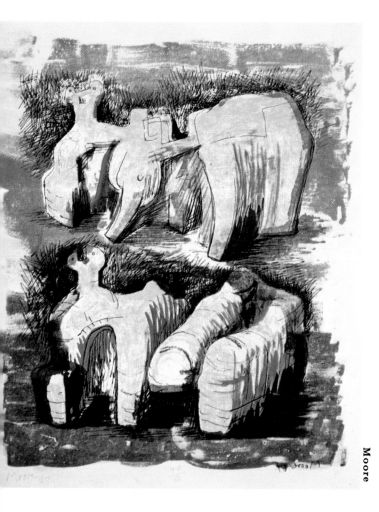

Moore

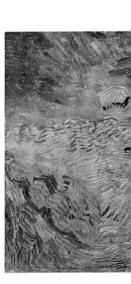

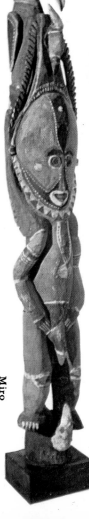

Miro

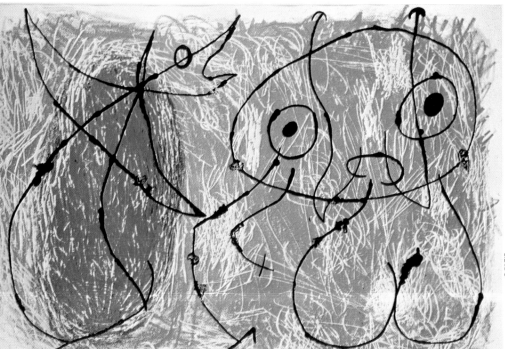

60

MARTHA "sits alone and cries. She wants
to get close to people but she finds it
hard to express her feelings because
she is afraid of being hurt." Her lack of
mouth and ears might show how hard it
really is for her to talk and listen.

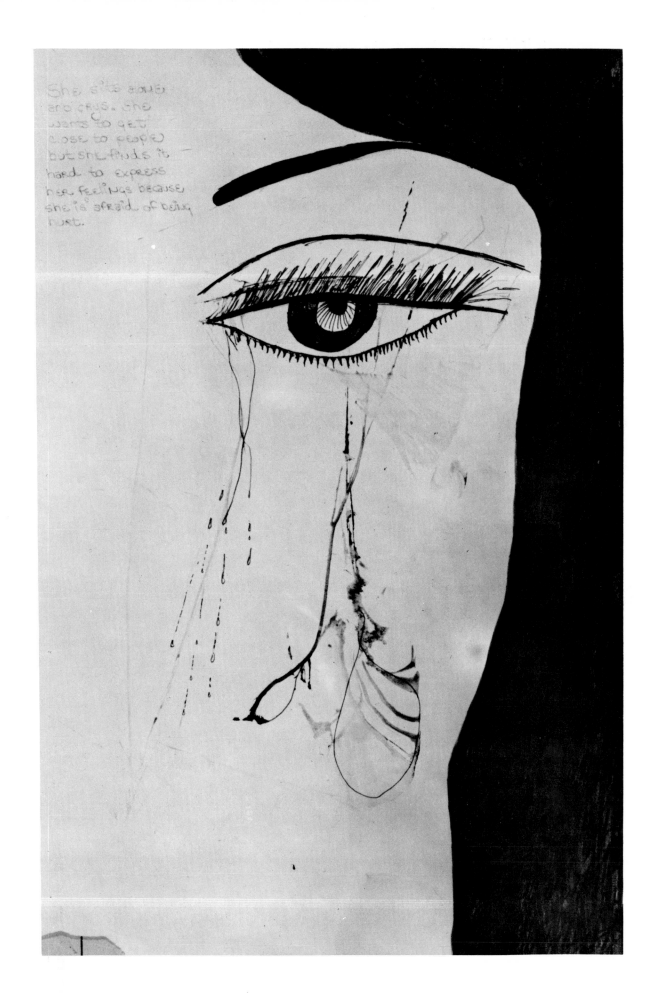

She sits alone
and cries. she
wants to get
close to people
but she finds it
hard to express
her feelings because
she is afraid of being
hurt.

61

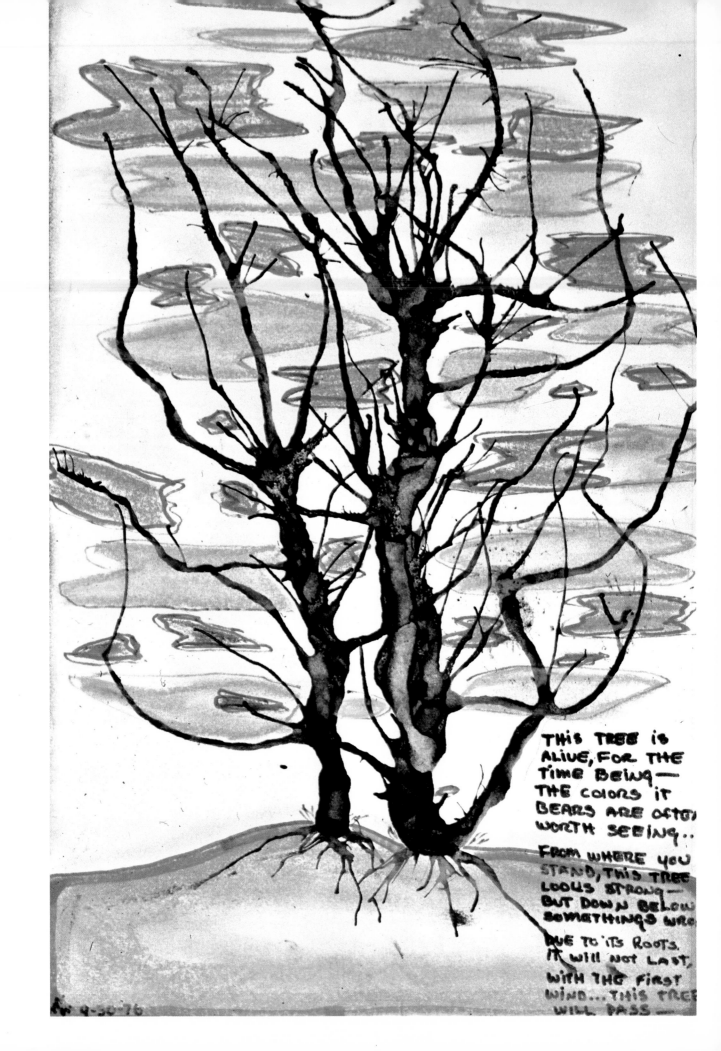

THIS TREE is
ALIVE, FOR THE
TIME BEING —
THE COLORS IT
BEARS ARE OFTEN
WORTH SEEING...

FROM WHERE YOU
STAND, THIS TREE
LOOKS STRONG —
BUT DOWN BELOW
SOMETHINGS WRONG.

DUE TO ITS ROOTS
IT WILL NOT LAST,
WITH THE FIRST
WIND... THIS TREE
WILL PASS —

62

One of the dimensions of art therapy is that it can promote the ability to relate and to communicate feelings in groups. The following experiences can help a heterogenous group of people understand and improve their interpersonal relationships through their artwork.

The first exercise is designed to allow each member of the group to share individually with the group. Ask the participants to draw their initials very large on a 14 by 17 paper. In the separate spaces created within or between the lines of the letters, have them draw something about themselves, about what they like to do, or about themselves and their families, that they may feel like sharing with the group. Ask them to hold their drawings up and tell the group what they have chosen to draw. No interpretations are needed. It is an easy way to establish contact, and gives everyone a few moments to hold forth about themselves.

Another way to encourage sharing individual feelings is to create a mask-making activity. Have the participants make a mask on one side of a paper bag about who they think they are. When

TOM wrote: "A vicious person dies and nobody can think of anything good to say about him on his tombstone. Nothing grows on the ground where he rests. Maybe God can see something good in you. I hope so."

TOM spent several years in prison and had lost contact with his children. He felt much abused and helpless.

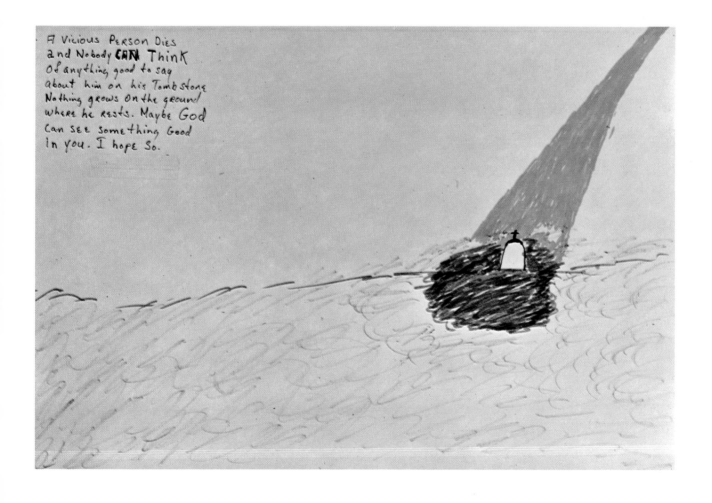

they are finished, have them make a mask on the other side of the bag of how they want to be. Supply scissors, colored paper, wool and other collage materials to facilitate the activity. Ask them to role-play, wearing their masks, play-acting the person they want to be. The experience of trying new behavior, with feedback from the group as they perform, helps them get a better idea of how they are perceived by others. The focus on the artwork gives enough distance so that they can become aware of parts of themselves without the anxiety of feeling that they are revealing too much.

The next exercise joins people in pairs drawing together silently, sharing space on one piece of paper for each pair. They are told to be aware of how they draw with each other, especially about sharing space, and how they feel if their lines cross or are crossed. After several nonverbal minutes, each pair tells the entire group about their experiences. During this exercise they often become aware that their own unique way of relating is not the only possible way for themselves or for others, and that how they feel about others crossing their

MOLLY was overweight. She was painfully honest with herself, but her masochism didn't seem to change her behavior. It did prevent people from telling her the same things, and from her being able to hear them.

She wrote: "This is my self-image at this time — a big blown-up fat body with no face — because I haven't found what my real face is yet."

64

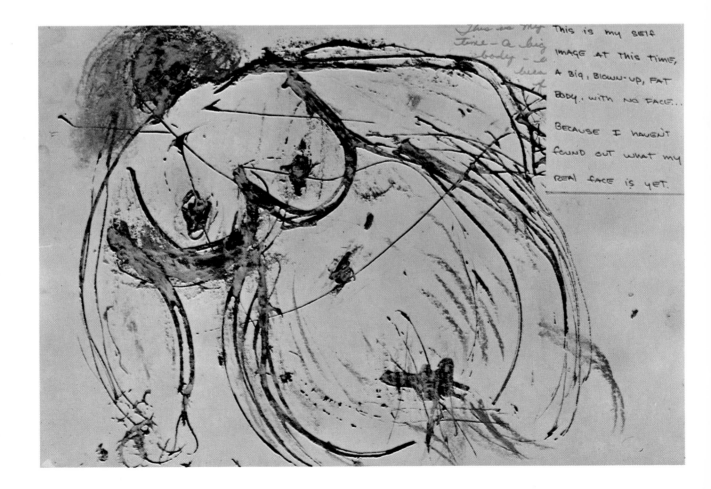

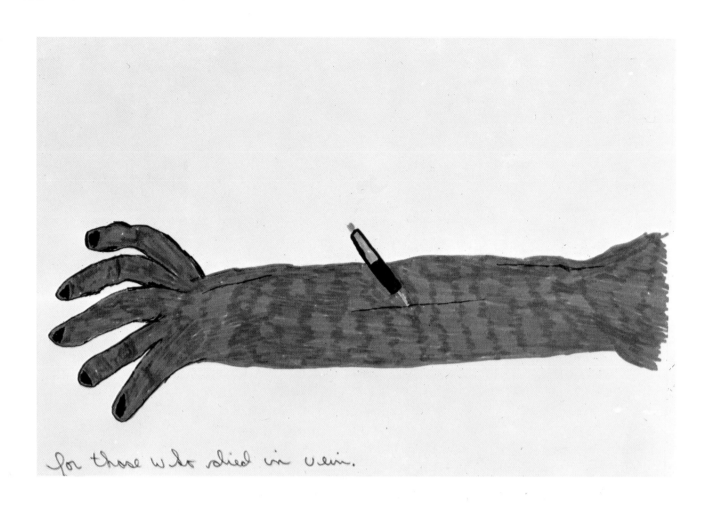

for those who died in vein.

lines or altering their pictures, or moving into their space and vice versa, can be compared with the way others feel about the experience.

This exercise can be a powerful learning experience. I recommend that it be repeated several times with different sets of partners to allow for the awareness of different personal styles and to give time and space for people to alter their own styles if they wish. All this learning takes place on a largely non-verbal level, experientially, and because of this has a powerful and lasting effect. The experience can be repeated in trios, allowing for an even larger range of behavior.

The next exercise is done in groups of five or six. Each person draws a picture for about three minutes, and then passes it to the right. Then each person draws on the neighbor's drawing, again for three minutes, and again passes it to the right, on and on until the original drawings have returned to the original artists. The discussion which follows may include feelings about spontaneity, about having their artwork altered, and about touching other people's work. The discussion can go in many directions, but what is even more important than what the feelings are is that the participants talk about their feelings, and discover it is O.K. to do so. They discover that they can listen to others talk, knowing they will have a turn, and that people really just want to say how they feel, don't really want advice, but just want to be heard and ac-

knowledged. Having shared feelings, the group can grow closer and more accepting of each other. In a low anxiety situation, with the focus on the artwork and not on them personally, they can learn how to share many feelings, even anger and hurt, with acceptance.

GROUP EXPERIENCE

A small group experience for six to eight people which can last several sessions, is that of doing a mural of a town. First the participants individually plan and create their own "model" towns. Then through discussion and compromise, a basic outline is jointly agreed on, and people assign themselves to draw different buildings of the town, while checking with their potential neighbors and accomodating to each other's needs. A great deal of non-verbal learning takes place while the participants develop the patience and understanding that it takes for groups to work together. Again, a lot of needs and feelings are displaced onto the kinds of buildings the people choose to focus on....food stores, amusement parks, fire stations, schools and other important parts of town, while the use of color helps to discharge feelings about these needs.

65

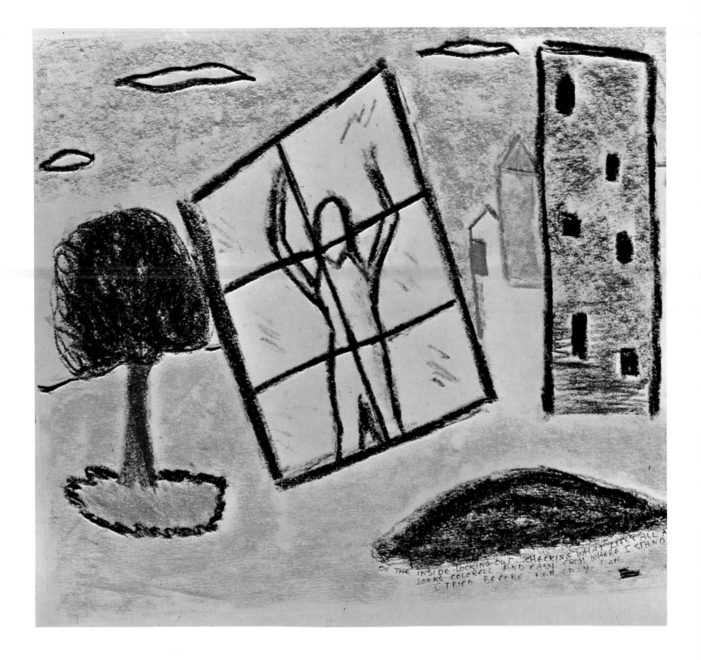

CREATING A SAFE SPACE

Our final group activity allows for a great deal of freedom by being laid in "space". In a furniture-less room, with butcher paper spread on the floor, the shoeless participants are told to choose an area of "space" and with the felt-tipped pens and oil pastels create their own individual worlds. When they have finished creating their space fantasies, they are free to visit one another. Make it a rule, however, that they have to ask permission of whomever they wish to visit, and create their own graphic means of transportation as they crawl across the paper. The permissive structure of this exercise and the feeling of space encourages inventiveness, and an expanded awareness of personal space. Non-verbal role modelling by the more creative and adventurous can help the less assertive people try new behavior as the people establish their territories on paper.

"On the inside looking out
Checking what life's all about
Looks colorful and easy
From where I stand.
I tried before and only ran."

The young poet seems to have framed and isolated himself from the colorful and easy life.

66

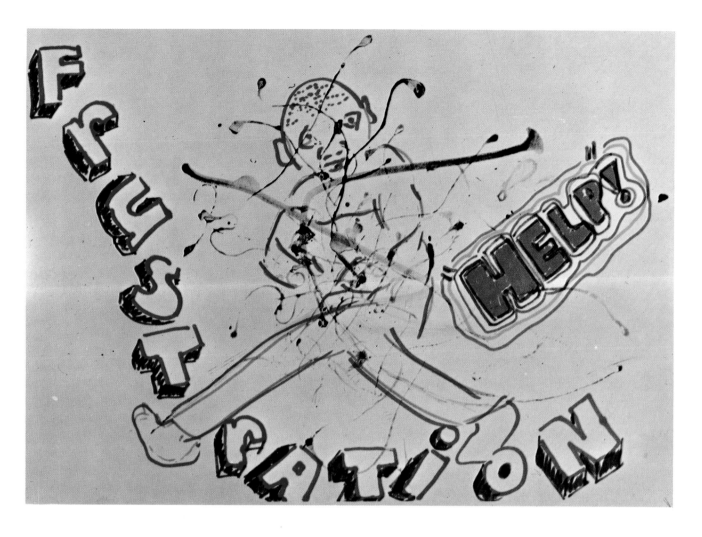

I was unable to locate the young man who drew this. The prognosis by the other patients was not good. They felt that he was either dead of an overdose or in jail.

PERCEPTION

It is important that at the end of each of these experiences, each of the participants have the opportunity to express some of the feelings about their perception of the activity if they wish to, so that a feeling of closure is established. The group can be encouraged to say what they have liked, haven't liked, what they might have learned about themselves and others, and any other ideas they might have for future games using art materials. It is not necessary for the leader to do more than encourage participation in the talk. It is sufficient to create the environment in which to work with the art materials and to allow the group to absorb themselves in the whole experience. The process of art will do the rest.

67

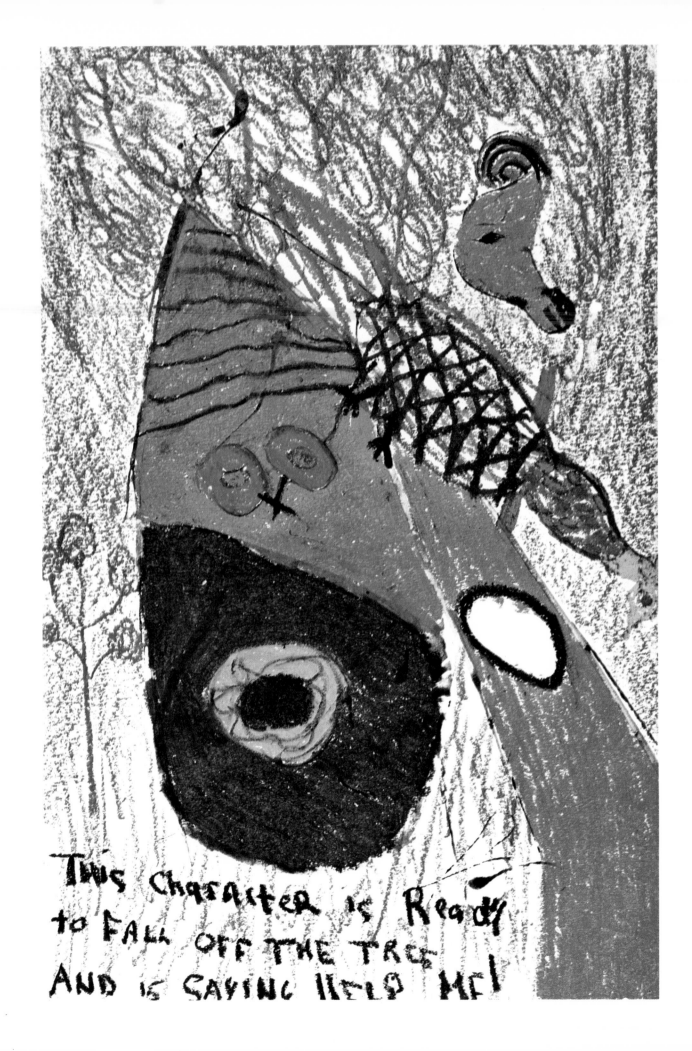

This Character is Ready
to FALL OFF THE TREE
AND is SAYING HELP ME!

These words demonstrate the powerless-
ness and general helplessness that the
patients all felt.

5.

drawing out my feelings

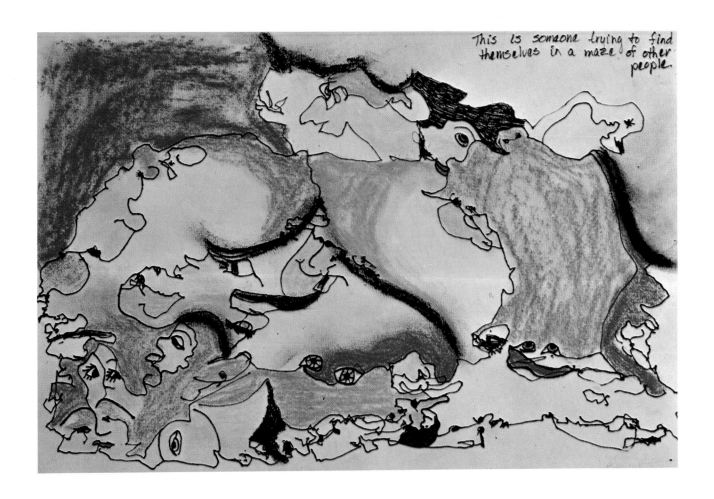

This is someone trying to find themselves in a maze of other people.

DONNA drew her first drawing shortly after she left the detoxification program and joined the rehabilitation program. She wrote: "This is someone trying to find themselves in a maze of other people." Her sense of self was lost in confusion.

When DONNA grasped the concept of art therapy, she threw herself into it and was much admired by the other patients for her inventiveness. She had been a runaway at age 16, working at odd jobs, and as a cocktail waitress.

She drew several women facing backwards, and considered the possibility that she was struggling with really looking inside and facing herself.

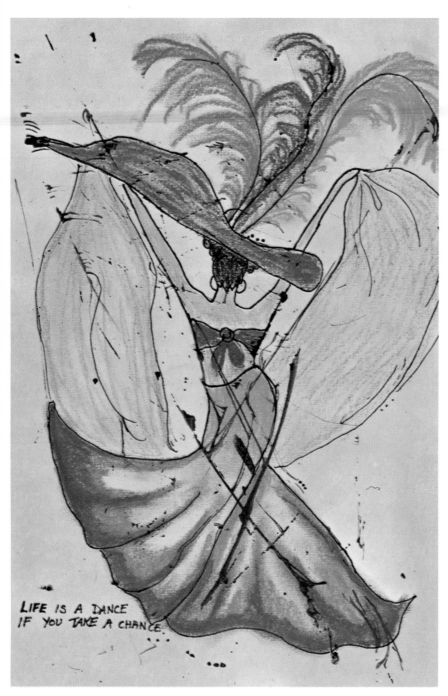

LIFE IS A DANCE
IF YOU TAKE A CHANCE.

72

Art therapy techniques can help us explore a then compare with each other how we experien and see the world. This allows us permission to ourselves and yet relate better to others who m see things differently. It lets us deal with the co flicting desires to be individual and yet part of t group.

One of the activities that lends itself well to t is problem-solving. The following exercise w developed originally for the mind's eye, by Jose Shorr in Psycho-Imagination Therapy.

Exercise I

Close your eyes and fantasize a chasm. Desi a way of crossing that chasm, considering that y have any and every means known or ev unknown as yet at your disposal. Draw your so tion and share it with the group.

Observe the solutions silently. Note the vario sizes of the chasms (problems) and the inve tiveness, efficiency and safeness of the vario solutions. If it is a rope bridge, is it tied securely? it is a huge chasm, is that how the person fe about his problem? Was the solution reached w little thought, or given a great deal of consider tion? If it is easily spanned, does that reflect th artist's ability to problem-solve?

By observing nonjudgmentally, all the artis will see for themselves the many ways of looking the same problem. In a safe environment, they c reach new conclusions, and if they like, adapt ne more varied ways of coping with problems. The is no one right way to cross a chasm ....there a as many ways as there are people, and some wa may seem to appear more effective than others

Roberto Assagioli in "Psychosynthes developed the following directed fantasy.

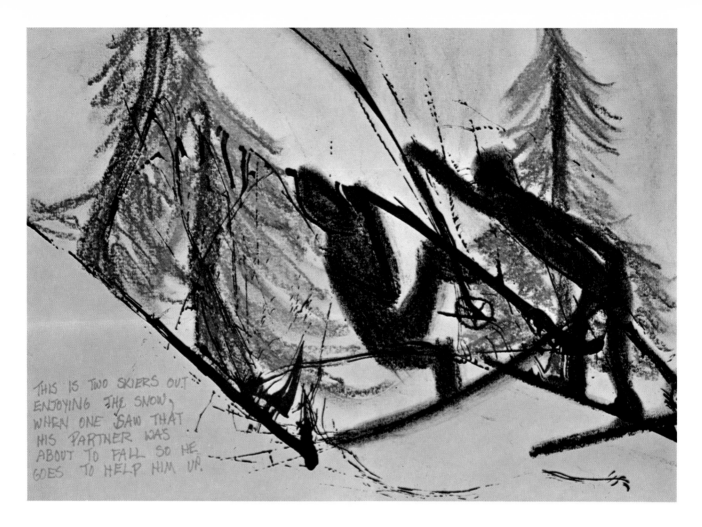

THIS IS TWO SKIERS OUT ENJOYING THE SNOW, WHEN ONE SAW THAT HIS PARTNER WAS ABOUT TO FALL SO HE GOES TO HELP HIM UP.

Exercise II

Fold a large piece of paper into quarters. Silently draw on the first quarter a symbolic representation of "WHERE DO I COME FROM?". After a few moments, draw on the second quarter, "WHERE DO I WANT TO GO?" Next draw symbolically "WHAT IS IN MY WAY?", and finally, "HOW AM I GOING TO OVERCOME MY OBSTACLES?"

Following this experience, those who wish to share, may, and those who wish to remain silent, may also. Be aware of how many people seem to hold others responsible for their own fears, sometimes realistically and at other times unrealistically. Young people, of course, experience the element of parental and teacher control, but with some, this is internalized and felt more powerfully than with others. This exercise can be a very moving experience and needs delicate or no intervention.

When people are asked to fantasize various situations with closed eyes, eidetic images, symbolic metaphors in our mind's eye, similar to dream images, appear. If we draw these and look at them as extensions and parts of ourselves, being aware of the use of color and line, we have another royal road to our unconscious to help us understand how we perceive the world and behave the ways that we do. One such experience which allows people to draw how they perceive the world is that of taking a fantasy trip with closed eyes.

DONNA was told by the others in the art therapy group that it appeared to them that the figure on the right was knocking the other figure down. We talked about the possibility that part of her was very resistant to being helpful to the part of her that wanted to give up her addiction.

73

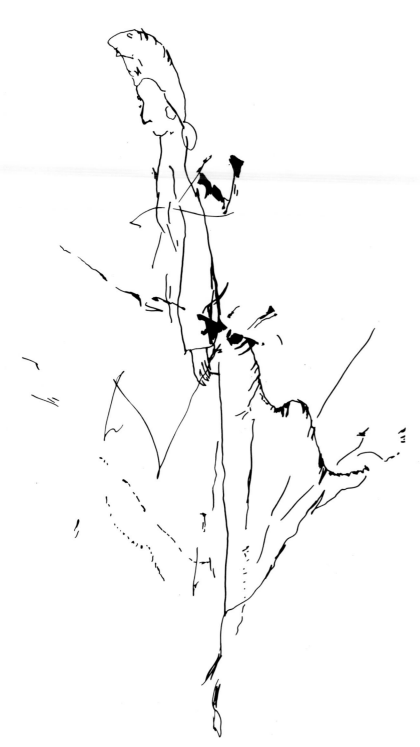

The line drawing was abandoned when she realized it was going to be an undressing figure. She did not want to deal with her shame of prostituting herself for drugs at the time so she turned the paper over.

Exercise III

Walking along a country road with a fishing pole, you come upon a stream. Cast a line into the water and after a few moments, reel in what you have caught in your fantasy. With your eyes open, draw what you have caught. Now write a story about the object at the end of the line. In a sense you will be talking about yourself and how you are feeling about your life at the moment. How do you see yourself?

These exercises are just a beginning. I have listed several books filled with inventive fantasy trips, many of which can be captured graphically, with line and color, adding another dimension to awareness. Art therapy can be nondirective, as when the individual projects forms onto an essentially formless background, as originally suggested by Leonardo Da Vinci, and then takes responsibility for the projection as representing aspects of himself, as suggested by Fritz Perls in Gestalt Therapy; or the exercise can be directed and task oriented, designed to bring out specific behaviors and feelings.

But we can also use others' creations to see what we will in them. Even looking at existing paintings and sculpture, and imagining being the persons, scenes or moods depicted, and making up stories about how we feel as those images will reveal more aspects of our complex personalities.

Also, paints and pastels are not the only materials to be used. Clay lends itself to nondirective art therapy beautifully. The feel alone of the plastic material is enough to produce many feelings and images. The use of clay, modelled with closed eyes, in silence, is a very effective way to become aware of one's self.

74

Then DONNA drew what looked like a coffin to her, writing, "Going to the door, she wants to leave....but what lurks in the darkness outside?" She added the lines to make the door and associated her drawing with her reluctance to stay in the program, and her fear of her addictive habits outside.

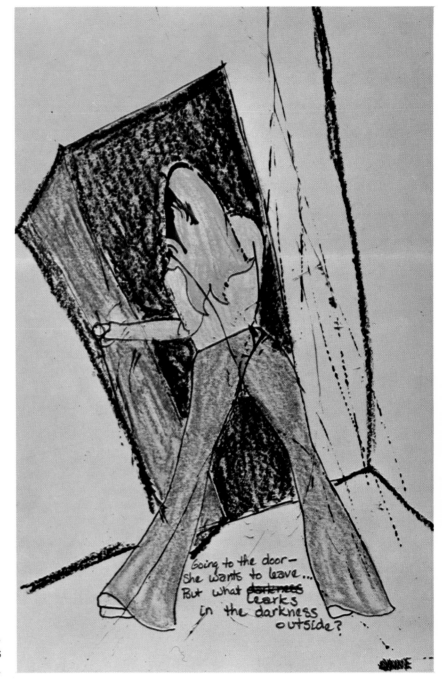

Exercise IV

As you feel the clay and squeeze, pound, jab, caress, or do what you wish to it; consider that this material is really you. Say to yourself, this is me, this is how I am feeling now. Spend ten to fifteen minutes experiencing the power of clay with no goals, no coiled pots, no ash trays or other goals in mind, just silently feeling the clay with eyes closed. Then study the form with open eyes for some new images to suggest themselves. If you intuitively become aware of a glimmer of an image, grasp it, and develop it. This is your metaphoric mind speaking to you.

These exercises will help unfold us to ourselves, and release our creativity if we allow them. Without expectations, "shoulds", without "ought to's"; just paying attention to our inner voices in a quiet environment will permit our fantasies to roam and will allow us to experience another side of ourselves, the hidden, rich, meditative, receptive side, which in the busy everyday world gets little attention.

DONNA told me that when she was lonely she would use heroin to make her "feel cuddled."

She said she would daydream a lot to avoid facing the pressures at the hospital. Her reputation as an artist grew, however, and she was given the responsibility to paint a large mural in the detoxification ward, to cheer up the patients. She was able to do a magnificent job.

DONNA finally turned around and began to draw herself out, figuratively and literally. She had been reluctant to smile much because her front teeth were cracked from having been beaten up frequently.

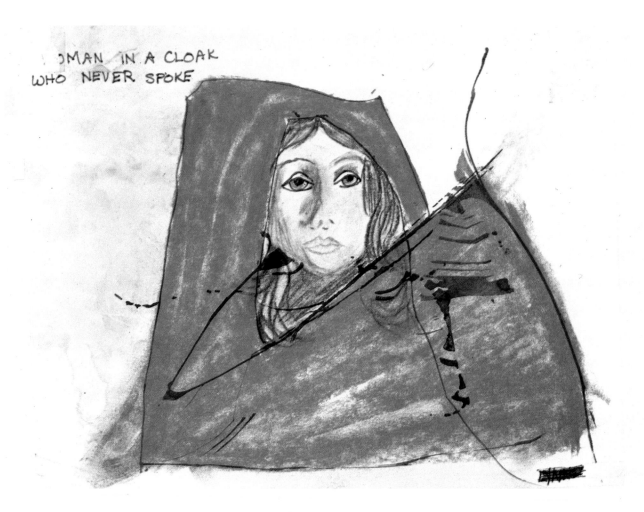

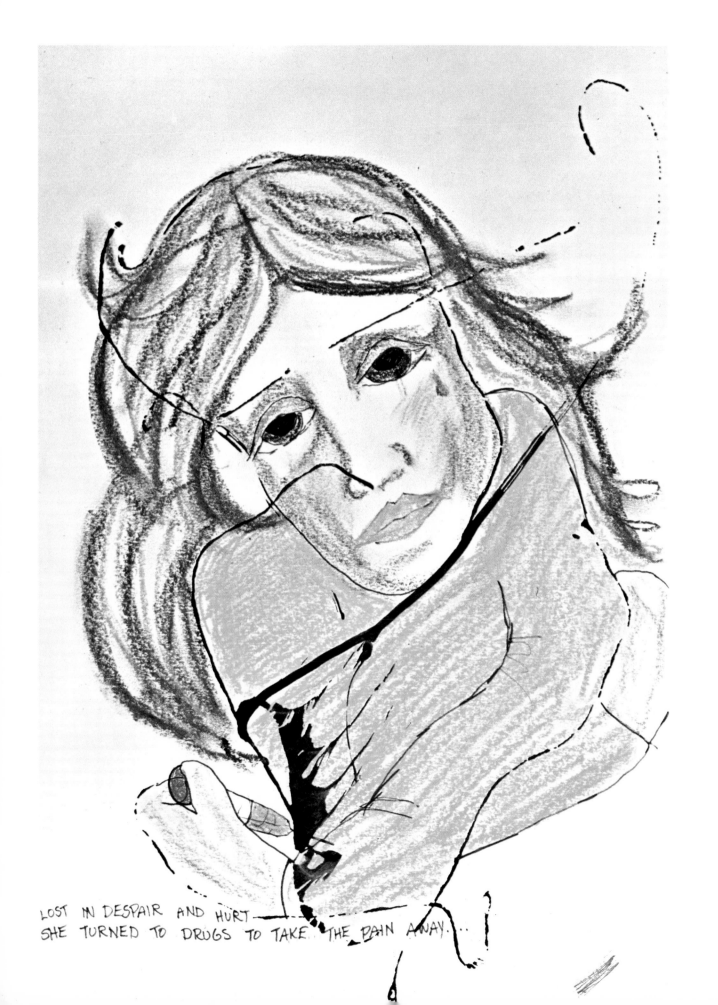

LOST IN DESPAIR AND HURT
SHE TURNED TO DRUGS TO TAKE THE PAIN AWAY...

9-2-76

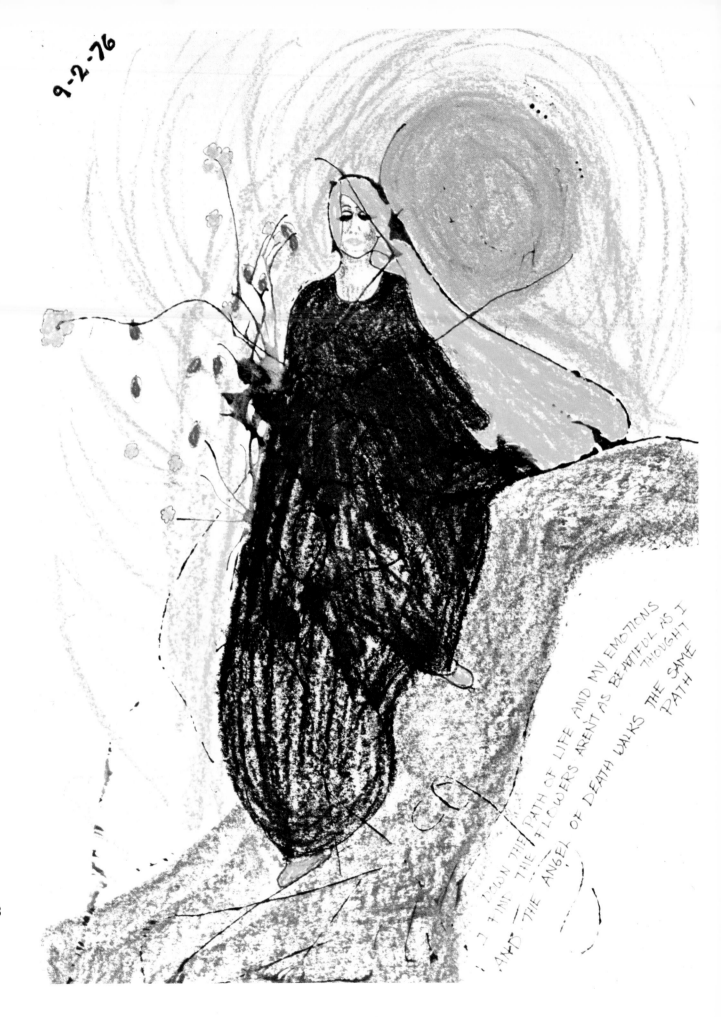

UPON THE PATH OF LIFE AND MY EMOTIONS
I FIND THE FLOWERS ARENT AS BEAUTIFUL AS I
THOUGHT
AND THE ANGEL OF DEATH WALKS THE SAME
PATH

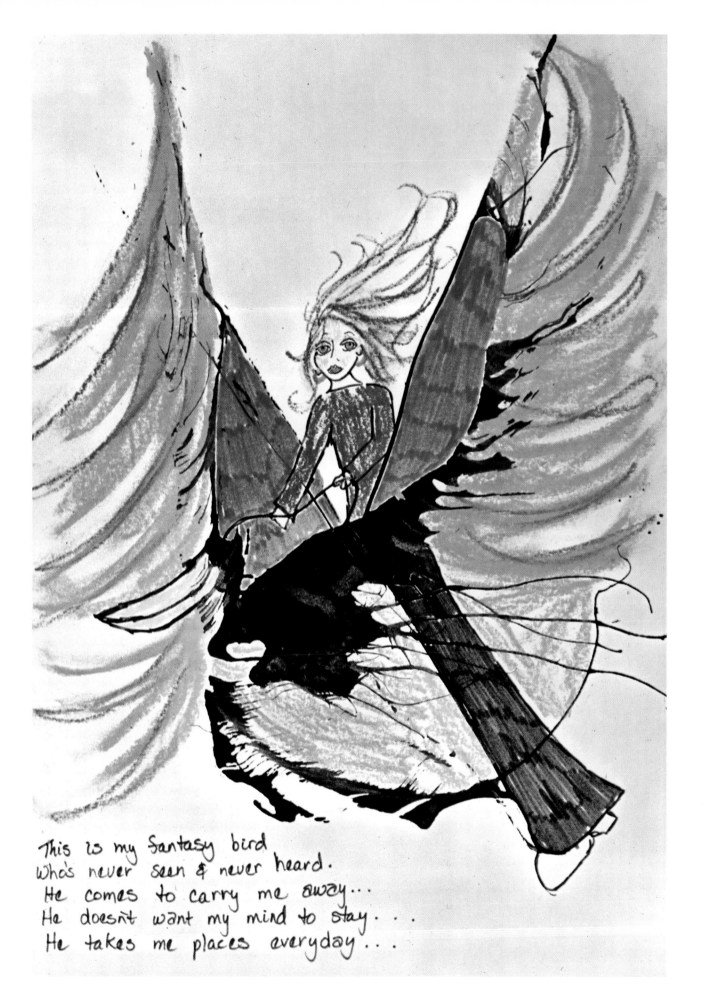

This is my fantasy bird
Who's never seen & never heard.
He comes to carry me away...
He doesn't want my mind to stay...
He takes me places everyday...

79

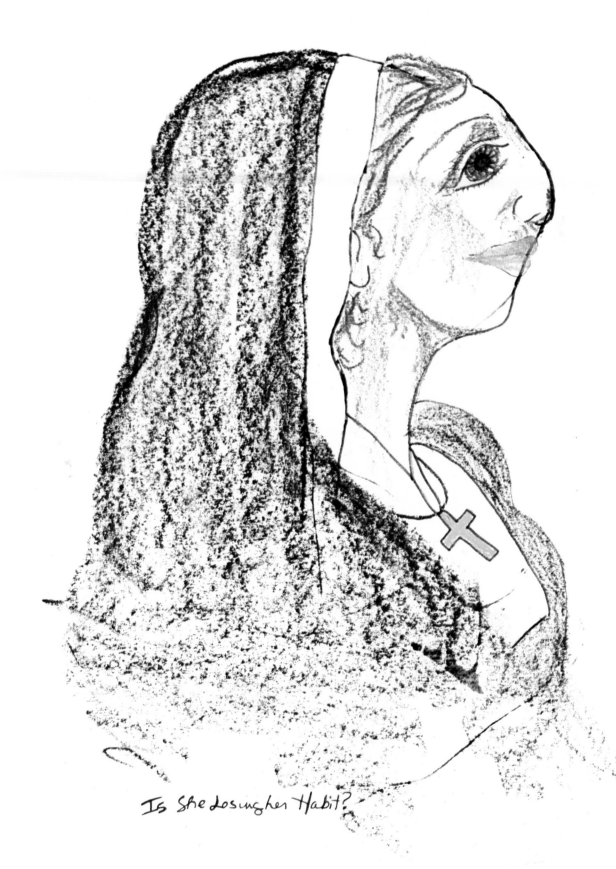

80

Is She Losing her Habit?

Donna's last drawing was done a week before she prematurely left the hospital against advice. She wrote, "Is she losing her habit?" When I last heard from her she had given up working as a cocktail waitress, had taken a job in a mill, and was, after 14 months, still off drugs.

6.

drawing to a close

The butterfly seems to be struggling, as was
the artist.

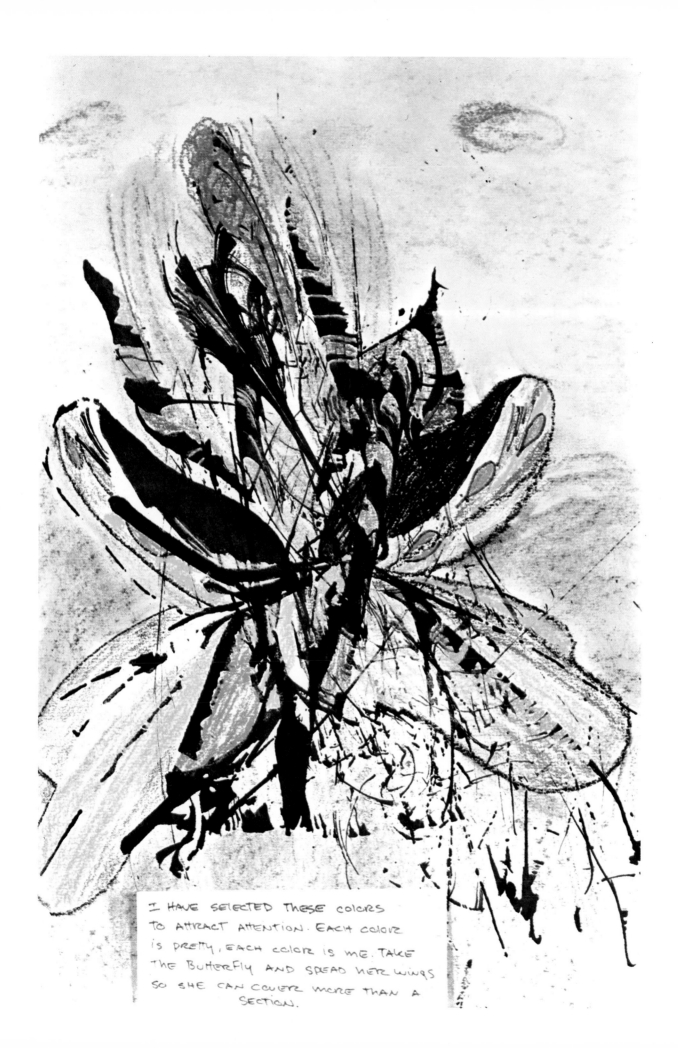

I HAVE SELECTED THESE COLORS
TO ATTRACT ATTENTION. EACH COLOR
IS PRETTY, EACH COLOR IS ME. TAKE
THE BUTTERFLY AND SPREAD HER WINGS
SO SHE CAN COVER MORE THAN A
SECTION.

83

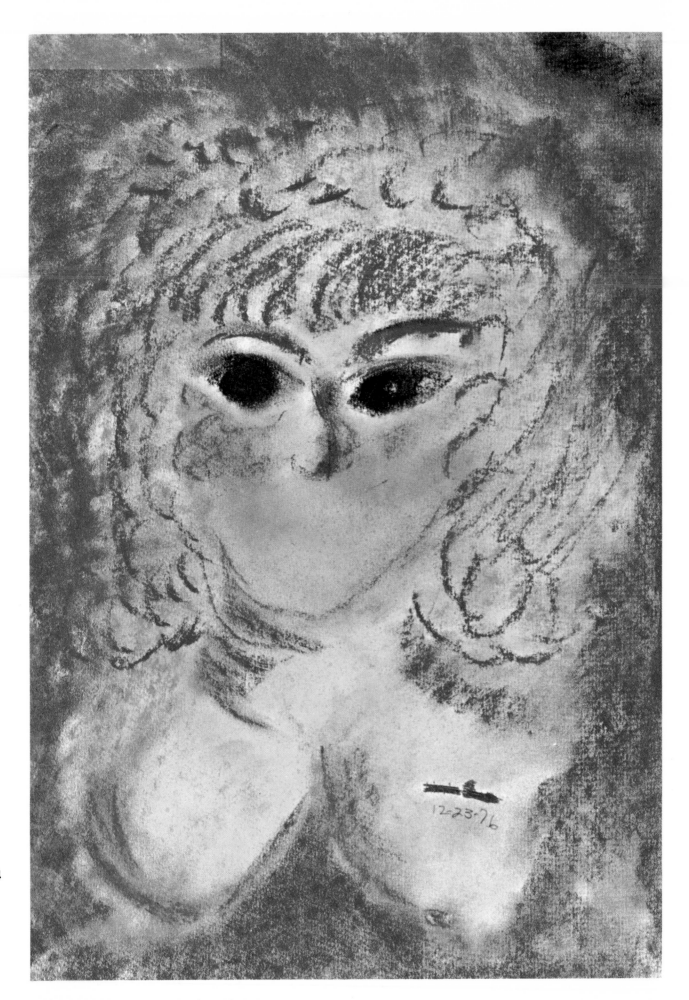

84

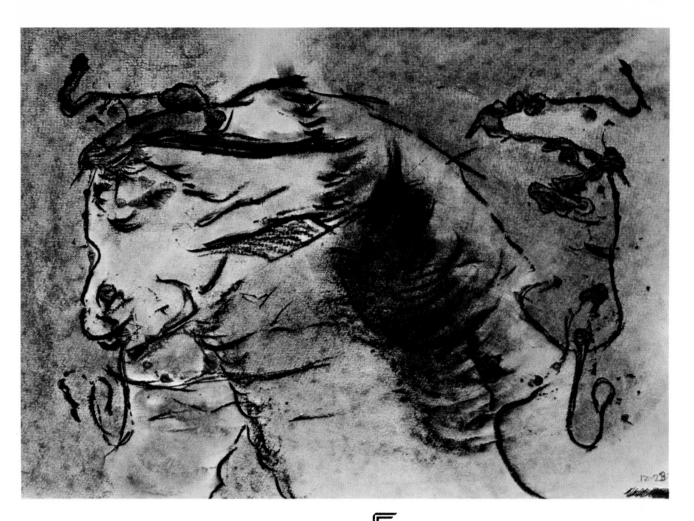

LORRAINE was silent as she worked on her first drawing in Art Therapy. She wrote a long paragraph about what the colors meant to her, and what the lack of mouth and the nippleless breasts meant. We talked about her jumbled words and finally I began to understand what she was saying, in the picture and the paragraph.

LORRAINE felt unable to express herself properly, because when she expressed warm feelings to people, she was taken advantage of sexually. She had decided that she was better off not talking...then she wouldn't get into trouble. But her drawing of her breasts suggests that perhaps she sometimes was responsible for what befell her.

After LORRAINE and I talked, she drew this most powerful horse, and wrote of her relief at having been able to explore her feelings about being helpless and feeling used and powerless.

Classically, art has been taught with a strong emphasis on form, perspective, color theory, design and other technical skills. Students who didn't absorb this technical information or who didn't "draw well" were labelled "untalented" or "uncreative" and were encouraged to develop other resources and pursue other interests.

I have been meeting many of these "untalented" students in their later years; they tremble with fear at the sight of a blank piece of paper and crayons, and they have an acute sense of inadequacy. Many of these people did indeed successfully pursue other interests and develop other resources and are leading "normal" lives, but to me they talk of feeling incomplete, unfinished, of missing something important in their lives. Others were not even this fortunate; they were unable to develop resources, and became failures in our society. Among these latter are, for example, drug addicts, losers in our society, with little education, no self-esteem, and self-destructive to the point of suicide. When I worked with these people for a year at the rehabilitation hospital, I found that given the non-evaluative opportunity to express their feelings with felt-tipped pens and pastels, they produced these most poignant, unique and powerful drawings. When asked to write poems or fantasies about their work, they were able to communicate some very powerful verbal expressions of feelings as you have seen.

85

When there were no goals or product orientation from the artistic point of view, merely a place where whatever marks they made on the paper were O.K.; when the only demand made of them was that they write something about what they had drawn; when there was no expectation of realism, rationality or neatness; then they expressed themselves, possibly for the first time in their lives; and they did so with imagination, openness, and effectiveness; and also possibly for the first time in their lives, self-respect.

I think that much current teaching of art involves techniques which favor the systematic, structured, cognitive functions, the so-called "left brain" functions. However, there are many people who are largely "right brain"; that is, they deal more in fantasy, intuition, movement, intangibles. Very often they daydream a lot, and may seem impractical. It is, of course, important for them to learn left-brain values and techniques, but they must also be validated and reinforced for the type of person that they are! Then, when they are allowed to express themselves non-directively, they can take pride in their creations and themselves. If you are confused and dismayed when confronted by what seems a formless scrawl, ask "What does this mean to you? What do you see in it?" And listen with admiration at the marvelous inventiveness and creativity of these "right-brain people"

You may only be giving them their lives.

CYNTHIA, a 20 year old clerical worker, born in Brentwood and the daughter of a successful businessman, has spent much time since age 13, in and out of psychiatric hospitals struggling with drugs and alcohol. She seems to accept responsibility for her addiction verbally, but she also acts like she has no power to stop herself.

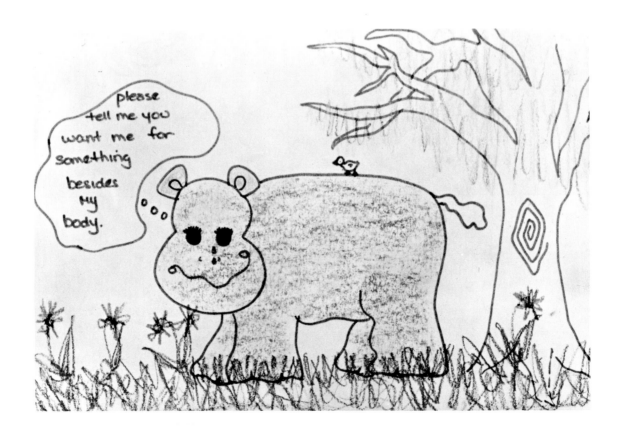

"Language", writes Arthur Koestler in THE ACT OF CREATION, "can become a screen which stands between the thinker and reality. This is the reason that true creativity often starts where language ends."

However, there are many language skills available to help the artist translate the graphic feelings about reality and creativity into words and understanding. That is part of what art therapy is about. To people, who may be interested in pursuing more information about art therapy, I recommend several books. Carl Roger's ON BECOMING A PERSON, (Houghton Mifflin) explains beautifully and clearly how to create an atmosphere where feelings can be shared openly, in a humanistic, non-authoritarian environment.

Janie Rhyne, THE GESTALT ART EXPERIENCE, (Brooks/Cole) and Margaret Frings Keyes, THE INWARD JOURNEY, (Celestial Arts) both talk about the art therapy process, and different exercises to help demystify the process of art.

For fantasy exercises to which you add the additional dimension of art, I recommend AWARENESS by John Stevens (Real People Press), GO SEE THE MOVIE IN YOUR HEAD by Joseph Shorr, (Popular Library), Richard De Mille's PUT YOUR MOTHER ON THE CEILING (Viking Compass), Kenneth Koch's WISHES, LIES AND DREAMS (Vintage) and EXPERIENCES IN VISUAL THINKING by Robert McKim, (Brooks /Cole).

I would like to share a quote with you in closing.

"I cannot forbear to mention . . . a new device for study which, although it may seem trivial and almost ludicrous, is nevertheless extremely useful in arousing the mind to various inventions. And this is, when you look at a wall spotted with stains . . . you may discover a resemblance to various landscapes, beautified with mountains, rivers, rocks, trees . . . or again you may see battles and figures in action, or strange faces and costumes and an endless variety of objects which you could reduce to complete and well-drawn forms. And these appear on such walls confusedly, like the sound of bells in whose jangle you may find any name or word you choose to imagine."

Leonardo Da Vinci, in his Notebooks

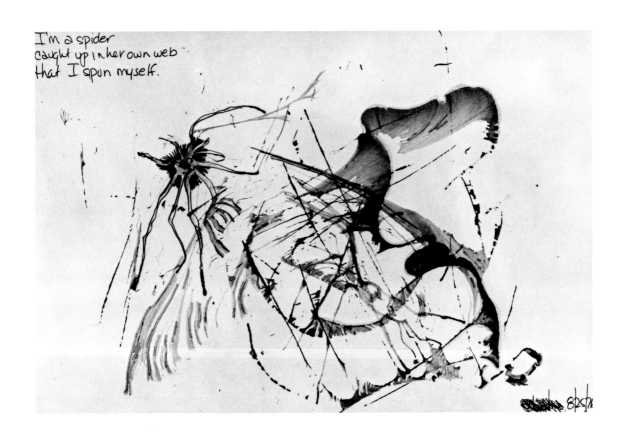

I'm a spider caught up in her own web that I spun myself.

87

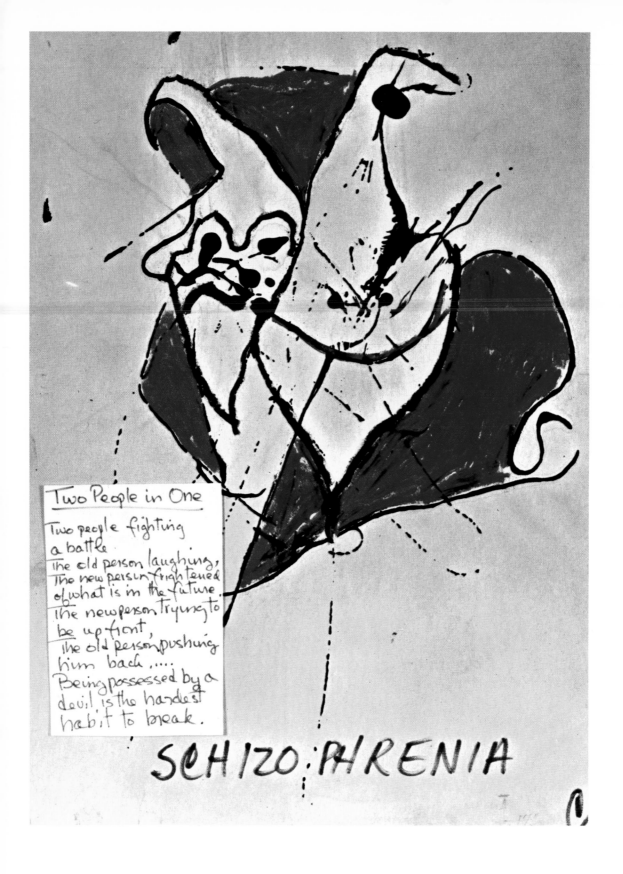

88

"A ghost who hid from himself and reality. He is lonely because he thinks people are afraid of him, but he is lovely." However, the word lovely looks like it originally was lonely. Most drug addicts at the hospital were very lonely when they entered, although many of them said they took drugs to "belong."

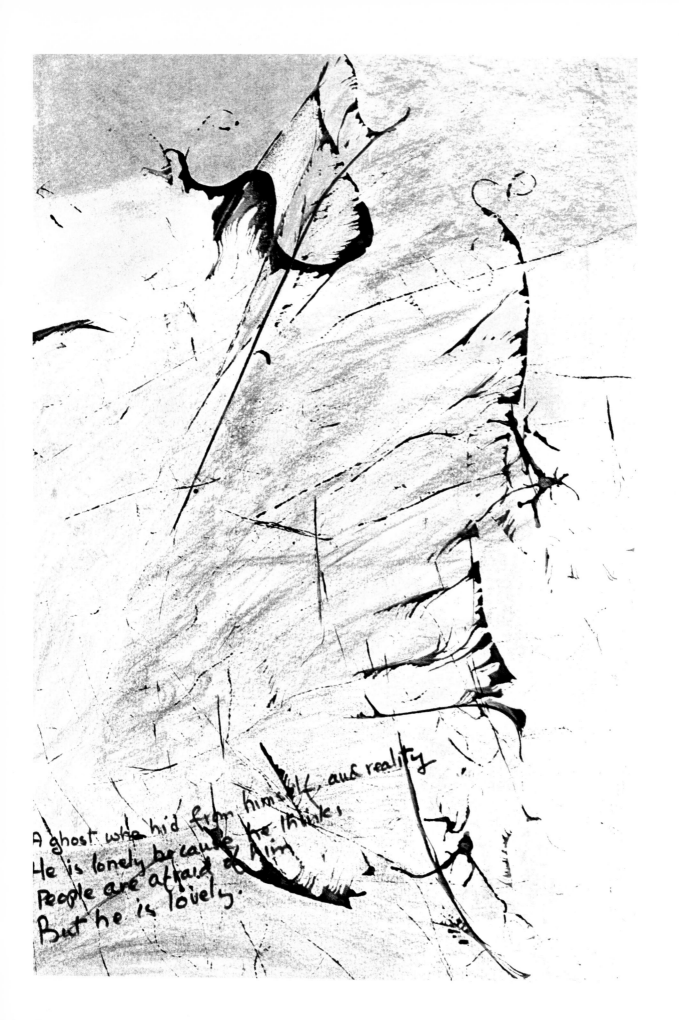

A ghost who hid from himself, and reality
He is lonely because he thinks
People are afraid of him
But he is lovely.

ANNA discovered the face inside after she
had completed her drawing. She wrote:
"Reaching out or being sucked in, which am
I?"

Her butterfly doesn't look like it can get off
the ground, although she sees it flying to the
sun.

90

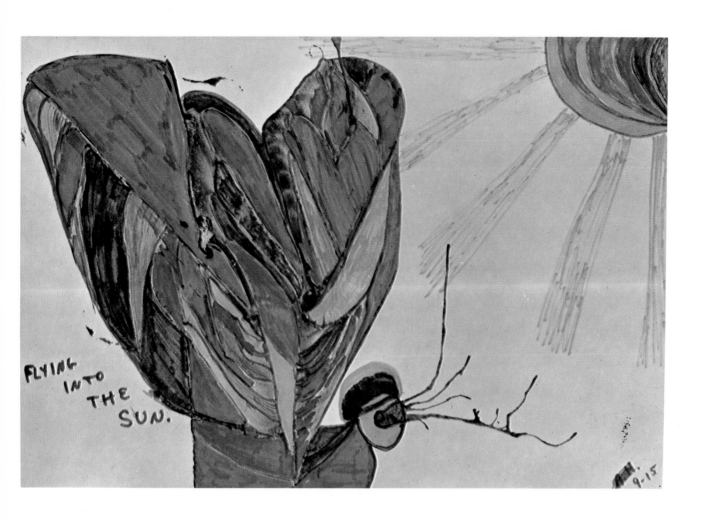

FLYING
INTO
THE
SUN.

BIRD WITHOUT
FEET, A BIRD
WITH HIS WINGS
TIED UP, I
FEEL VERY TIGHT,
CLOSED UP.

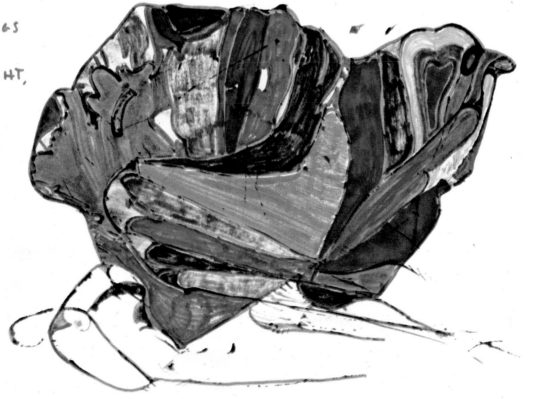

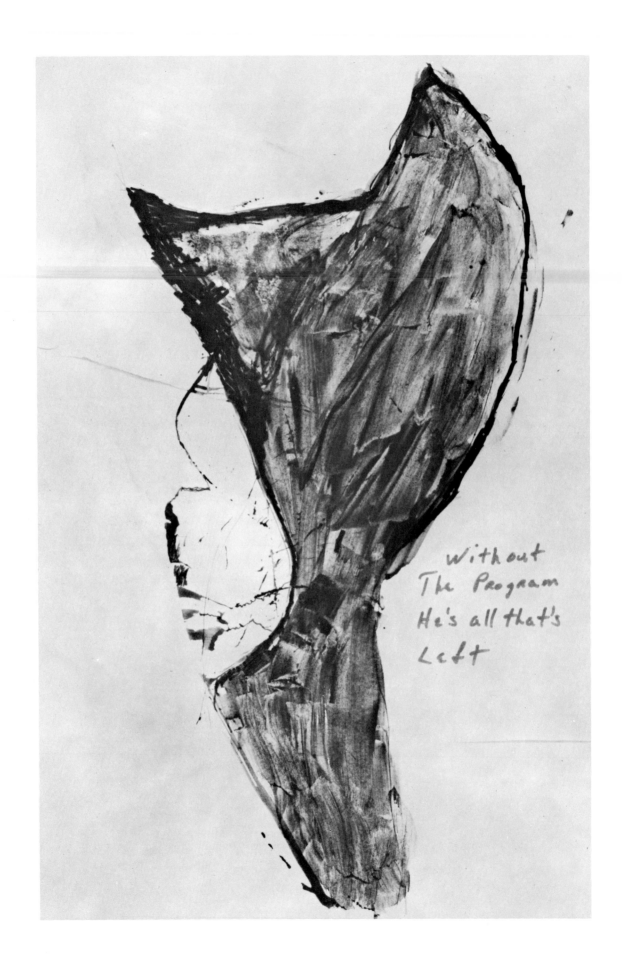

Without
The Program
He's all that's
Left

92

BIBLIOGRAPHY

ART THERAPY

Alshuler, R. and Hattwick, L.B., PAINTING AND PERSONALITY,
    Illinois: University of Chicago, 1969.

Axline, V., DIBS, IN SEARCH OF SELF, Boston: Houghton, 1964.

Barnes, M. and Berke, J., TWO ACCOUNTS OF A JOURNEY THROUGH MADNESS,
    New York: Ballantine, 1973.

Capacchioni, L., THE CREATIVE JOURNAL, Chicago: Swallow Press, 1978.

Keyes, M., THE INWARD JOURNEY, ART AS THERAPY FOR YOU,
    California: Celestial Arts, 1974.

Kramer, E., ART AS THERAPY WITH CHILDREN, New York: Schocken, 1971.

Milner, M., ON NOT BEING ABLE TO PAINT, New York: International University, 1973.

Naumberg, M., DYNAMICALLY ORIENTED ART THERAPY: ITS PRINCIPLES AND
    PRACTICE, New York: Grune and Stratton, 1966.
    AN INTRODUCTION TO ART THERAPY, New York: Teachers College,
    1973.

Prinzhorn, H., ARTISTRY OF THE MENTALLY ILL, New York: Springer-Verlag, 1972.

Rhyne, J., THE GESTALT ART EXPERIENCE, California: Brooks/Cole, 1974.

Rubin, J., CHILD ART THERAPY, New York: Van Nostrand Reinhold, 1978.

ART

Arguelles, J., THE TRANSFORMATIVE VISION, California: Shambhala, 1975.

Arguelles, J., and M., MANDALA, California: Shambhala, 1972.

Arnheim, R., THE GENESIS OF A PAINTING, California: University of California, 1969.

Cardinal, R., OUTSIDER ART, New York: Praeger, 1972.

Cockroft, E., Weber, J., and Cockroft, J., TOWARDS A PEOPLE'S ART,
    New York: Dutton, 1977.

Franck, F., THE ZEN OF SEEING/DRAWING, New York: Vintage Press, 1973.

Hill, E., THE LANGUAGE OF DRAWING, New Jersey: Prentice Hall, 1966.

Klee, P., ON MODERN ART, London: Curwen, 1969.

McKim, R., EXPERIENCES IN VISUAL THINKING, California: Brooks/Cole, 1972.

O'Brien, J., DESIGN BY ACCIDENT, New York: Dover, 1968.

Read, H., ART AND ALIENATION, New York: Viking, 1967
    THE MEANING OF ART, New York: Penguin, 1964

Rottger/Klante, CREATIVE DRAWING, New York: Van Nostrand Reinhold, 1963.

Stone, I., DEAR THEO, THE AUTOBIOGRAPHY OF VINCENT VAN GOGH, New York:
    Doubleday, 1937.

IMAGERY

De Mille, R., PUT YOUR MOTHER ON THE CEILING, New York: Viking, 1973.

Koch, K., WISHES, DREAMS AND LIES, New York: Vintage, 1971.

Masters, R., and Houston, J., MIND GAMES, THE GUIDE TO INNER SPACE, New York: Delta, 1972.

Samuels, M., and Samuels, N., SEEING WITH THE MIND'S EYE, New York: Random House, 1975.

Shorr, J., GO SEE THE MOVIE IN YOUR HEAD, New York: Popular Library, 1977.

Stevens, J., AWARENESS: EXPLORING, EXPERIMENTING, EXPERIENCING, California: Real People Press, 1971.

PSYCHOLOGY

Assagioli, R., PSYCHOSYNTHESIS, New York: Viking, 1971.

Bogen, J., THE OTHER SIDE OF THE BRAIN, Bulletin of the Los Angeles Neurological Societies, Vol. 34, July, 1969.

Bogen, J. E., and Vogel, P. J., CEREBRAL COMMISSUROTOMY IN MAN: MINOR HEMISPHERE DOMINANCE FOR CERTAIN SPATIAL FUNCTIONS, Journal of Neurosurgery, Vol. 23, 1962.

Freud, S., THE PLEASURE PRINCIPLE, ON DREAMS, New York: Norton, 1952.

Gazzaniga, M. S., THE BISECTED BRAIN, New York: Appleton-Century-Crofts, 1970.

Ghiselin, B., Ed., THE CREATIVE PROCESS, California: University of California, 1952.

Jaynes, J., THE ORIGIN OF CONSCIOUSNESS IN THE BREAKDOWN OF THE BICAMERAL MIND, Boston: Houghton Mifflin, 1976.

Jourard, S., THE TRANSPARENT SELF, Princeton: Van Nostrand, 1964.

Jung, C. G., MEMORIES, DREAMS AND REFLECTIONS, New York: Vintage, 1961, THE PORTABLE JUNG, New York: Viking, 1971, MAN AND HIS SYMBOLS, New York: Doubleday, 1969.

Laing, R. D., THE DIVIDED SELF, New York: Pantheon, 1969.

Maslow, A., TOWARDS A PSYCHOLOGY OF BEING, New York: Van Nostrand, 1968.

May, R., THE COURAGE TO CREATE, New York: Norton, 1965.

Ornstein, R., THE PSYCHOLOGY OF CONSCIOUSNESS, California: Freeman, 1972.

Perls, F., GESTALT THERAPY VERBATIM, California: Real People Press, 1969.

Rogers, C., ON BECOMING A PERSON, Boston: Houghton Mifflin, 1961.

Sagan, C., THE DRAGONS OF EDEN, New York: Random House, 1977.

Shorr, J., PSYCHOTHERAPY THROUGH IMAGERY, New York: IMBC, 1974.

Sperry, R. W., THE GREAT CEREBRAL COMMISSURE, Scientific American, Jan. 1964.

Von Franz, M. and Hillman, J., JUNG'S TYPOLOGY, New York: Spring, 1971.

Whitmont, E., THE SYMBOLIC QUEST, New York: Jung Foundation, 1969.

index

95